MAXIMUM FAT LOSS
WORKBOOK

TED BROER
AMERICA'S **MAXIMUM HEALTH** EXPERT

Published by B & A Publications

ISBN 0-7852-6735-2

Printed in the United States of America
5 6 VP 08 07

CONTENTS

TWELVE WEEKS TOWARD LEAN!

The seasons of the year are quarterly: spring, summer, autumn, and winter. The business world operates on a quarterly cycle. So do a number of universities, high school programs, and small-group studies. We seem intuitively programmed as human beings to think in terms of ninety-day cycles.

There's no real magic to a ninety-day time frame. There is however a great deal to be said for this time frame. A three-month period is just about right for revamping a long-standing habit, both mentally and physically. Many recovery centers (such as drug-rehab centers) are based on a twelve-week program. It takes a while for both body and mind to sync up into a new routine. The same is true for a fat-loss program.

A TWELVE-WEEK PROGRAM FOR FAT LOSS

Twelve weeks. Twelve changes. This workbook presents a new set of habits for pursuing fat loss until you reach your goal, and then maintaining your fat loss the rest of your life. That's what this book is all about.

You may not lose all the fat you desire to lose in twelve weeks, and that is certainly so if you are more than twenty-five pounds overweight. What you *will* do during this twelve-week period is begin to make the necessary changes—one change a week—to adjust the way you think about fat, as well as what you eat and drink, how and when you take supplements, and how and when you do what kinds of exercise in order to get lean and stay lean.

Again, this program calls for you to make just one change each week until you have fully implemented the complete fat-loss program. Most people find it easy to make one change at a time.

At the end of the twelve weeks, you should have implemented all of the changes, and the fat should be melting away from your body. The more changes you make, the more motivated you will feel toward implementation of the entire program. These twelve weeks are a duplicate of my clinically-tested fat-loss program that can and should become a lifelong habit for you.

Certainly if you desire to make all of the changes in the first week, you can do so. There's nothing at all to prohibit that physiologically or psychologically.

WHY ONLY ONE CHANGE A WEEK?

There's an old saying, "All emphasis is no emphasis." Too many times when we promise ourselves that we are going to change everything about the way we are living—or exercising, eating, and pursuing maximum fat loss—we change *nothing*. The task seems too monumental and we may stay on track for a few days, but when things become tedious or we don't see the progress we'd like to see, we drop the entire program and write it off as another try. That's why this program calls for you to change just one thing a week. By making a gradual transition to the new patterns of behavior that you seek to establish, you are more likely to adopt those new patterns of behavior until they become habit.

Keep in mind that you can *physically* change things sometimes far faster than you can change things *mentally*. I have met a number of people who tell me that even though they have lost twenty, thirty, forty, fifty pounds . . . they still *think* of themselves as being overweight. Even though they have lost a lot of fat, they still find themselves shopping for clothes to hide their fat. Even though they have been eating the right foods for weeks, even months, they still find choosing the right foods to be something of a daily struggle. The wrong foods are still a temptation!

Keep in mind that your current pattern of eating and exercise likely are deeply-ingrained *habits*. You automatically reached for certain foods, both in the grocery store and on your own pantry or refrigerator shelves, without much thought. You automatically *don't* exercise . . . To exercise now means a new level of intention and effort on your part. To change a habit at the physical level is one thing, but to change it in the *mind* is another. It may take a number of months, or even longer, for you to see yourself mentally as you really are: a lean, healthy, energetic person.

By taking just one step at a time, over a twelve-week period, you give your mind a chance to accommodate and to accept new patterns of living, as well as new patterns of thinking. Give your mind a chance to readjust, just as your body is readjusting to a new metabolic rate and a new set of routines.

AN OVERVIEW OF THE WEEKS AHEAD

Here's where we're headed on a week-by-week basis:

Week #1

This is your week for coming to a *commitment* that you are going to do whatever it takes to lose your excess fat.

If you have not already read my book, *Maximum Fat Loss*, I hope you will use the first week to do so. At about fifty pages a night (less than an hour of reading for most readers), you should be able to finish the book in a week. The book presents the basic concepts and underlying scientific information that is at the heart of the maximum fat loss program.

Week #2

In this week, you will be asked to undertake a complete physical appraisal—primarily an objective evaluation and documentation of what you weigh and your physical measurements. Then you will be asked to set a realistic goal as to how many calories you are going to consume daily.

Week #3

In this week, you will eat six meals a day with a total calorie count of ten times that of your ideal weight.

Week #4

This is your week to learn how to make a protein shake and to eat the right amount and right kinds of protein each day.

Week #5

This is your week to get your carbohydrates in balance with your protein and to choose the right carbohydrates: low-glycemic-index fruits and vegetables.

Week #6

This is the week to get fatty acids incorporated into your eating plan and to make sure that your daily protein, carbohydrate, and fat intake is in balance.

Week #7

This is pantry-cleaning week! It is the time to dump the sugar bowl and to completely eliminate all the "bad carbs" from your house.

Week #8

In this week, you will be asked to make certain that you are drinking sufficient water each day.

Week #9

This week you will be challenged to make sure your fiber intake is sufficient.

Week #10

You should already be exercising—this is your week to make certain you are well into the rhythm of doing twenty-five minutes of cardiovascular (aerobic) exercise five times a week.

Week #11

This is the week to make certain that you are doing flexibility (stretching) and strength-building (weights) exercises three to four times a week.

Week #12

This is the week to check your supplements and make sure you are taking in all the nutrients your body needs for maximum fat loss.

Each week you will also be asked to take very specific "Action Steps" that may not be directly related to the overall challenge of the week but that can put you on your way to establishing the eating and exercise habits you need to achieve maximum fat loss.

At the end of the twelve weeks you will have put together a complete plan for fat loss that culminates in a new daily schedule and periodic check-points for the months ahead.

If you feel you would like to make these changes more quickly than twelve weeks . . . go for it! Many of my clients implement the majority of these healthy choices the first week with outstanding, sometimes nearly miraculous, results.

OTHER ELEMENTS IN THIS BOOK

Interspersed throughout this workbook you will find three elements:

Questions to Consider

These thought-provoking questions give you an opportunity to explore more fully your own opinions about fat, fat loss, and your own desires to become lean and fit. Tackle only one question at a sitting. Give thoughtful reflection to the question and be honest with yourself. This is not a time to say what you think others might want you to say. This is your workbook—the answers you give should be for your eyes only, and for your own self-understanding.

Fat Facts

These tidbits present facts related to the harmful consequences associated with excess fat, the process of fat loss, and the things you can anticipate as you lose fat. These facts are presented not only to inform, but to encourage and motivate you in your fat-loss program.

Fat-Loss Tip

These tips are very practical and they can be incorporated at any time into your fat-loss program.

Forms to Chart Your Progress

You may want to purchase a three-ring binder so you can duplicate some of the forms and charts that are in this workbook and then continually update your progress as the weeks and months go by.

In all . . .

This is a book you *do* . . . not just a book you read. Get a sharp pencil and let's take the first step toward a lifetime of lean!

MORE THAN A COMMITMENT —A *DESIRE!*

WEEK #1

CHALLENGE AND CHANGE FOR WEEK #1
Develop a deep desire to do whatever it
takes to lose your excess fat.

FAT-LOSS TIP

Eat meals one hour after exercise.

Breaking the "Fat Patterns"

There seem to be three basic *mental* fat patterns that people acquire through the years:

1. bad information about fat and losing fat

2. bad eating habits

3. bad excuses for remaining fat

Again, these bad patterns are rooted in the mind. Before you can truly have a deep desire to do whatever it takes to lose your excess fat, you must come to grips with the reasons for why you haven't already lost your excess fat!

Bad Information

Too many people have bought into excuses about why they are fat and why they can't seem to lose weight and keep it off. Below is a sampling of these excuses I've heard.

Excuses about Fat and Fat Loss

- I'm a woman so I'm just naturally fatter. (You are genetically predisposed to carry more fat, but that doesn't mean you must be overfat!)

- I have a slow metabolism and metabolism can't be changed. (Very easy to fix.)

- I'm fat because my parents are fat—it's genetic. (Family dietary patterns are the primary cause of obesity . . . not genetics.)

- I was born with too many fat cells. (Not true. These cells develop within the first few years of life.)

- I've tried dieting but diets just never seem to work for me. (This book does not reflect a diet. Diets don't work. This is a lifeplan choice!)

- I have large bones and large-boned people automatically are fatter. (Large bones may make you bigger, but not fatter.)

- I'm not really fat . . . I'm just heavyset. (Right, and I'm the tooth fairy.)

- I've had babies so I have a fat stomach. (Your stomach may be stretched but exercise can help.)

- I'm too old now to do anything about losing fat—lean bodies are for the young. (Never true. Please don't put this attitude into concrete. It can kill you.)

- I've exercised before and the fat just doesn't go away—exercise doesn't work for me. (That's because eighty percent of how you look depends on how you eat.)

- Weight doesn't really matter—it's only who you are on the inside that counts. (That may be true from a personality standpoint, but fat also can drastically effect your health.)

- I may be significantly overweight, but I'm healthy. (I've never seen someone who is significantly overweight who is also healthy.)

Write down three of the biggest excuses you seem to have accepted into your life.

The Top Three Excuses about Fat and Fat Loss that I Have Accepted as Truth

1.

2.

3.

Now take your pen or pencil and draw a line through each of these statements you have written. In the margin to the right, write in large, bold letters: "EXCUSE!"

Instead of believing excuses about your own excess fat, choose instead to believe the truth. There's room below to write three positive, truthful statements you need to adopt as part of your new mental perspective on fat loss. Again, some sample statements have been provided for you.

THE TRUTH ABOUT FAT AND FAT LOSS

- I can lose my excess fat.

- I can change my metabolism through exercise.

- I can choose to have empty fat cells.

- What I do about filling or depleting my fat cells is up to me and nobody else.

- I am the person responsible for what I weigh and how much fat I have, and I am therefore also the person responsible for the fat I lose.

- I can adopt new patterns of eating and exercise that will work to reduce the percentage of fat in my body.

- Fat is not good for my health and I'm going to face that fact and do something about it.

- I can have a lean, fit body at my age.

- I may have large bones, but I do not need to accept excess fat!

- Excess fat does put limitations on my energy—I can lose fat and have more energy.

- Being fat does have an impact on my self-esteem—I can choose to lose fat and improve my own image of myself, even as I improve the image of my body.

- Fat loss may require consistency, but I'm a person who is capable of taking on challenges and accomplishing goals!

THE TRUTH ABOUT MY FAT

_____

_____

_____

_____

_____

_____

Now write next to each of the statements above a large, bold "YES!"

Bad Eating Habits

Many people have acquired bad eating habits through the years. Most _know_ these habits are bad. If you don't think you have bad eating habits and you are carrying excess fat, you simply haven't been informed about your habits! A number of my clients have come to me through the years knowing that diets haven't worked for them, but unsure as to why. They quickly discovered their bad habits by reading through the basic principles presented in _Maximum Fat Loss_.

Bad eating habits stand in a person's way as obstacles to fat loss, not necessarily at the physiological level, but at the _mental_ level.

Below are some of the habits my clients have admitted to me. Also below is your opportunity to identify at least five bad habits you know you need to change in order to achieve maximum fat loss and maintain that fat loss the rest of your life.

BAD EATING HABITS THAT NEED CHANGING

- Too much of our family cooking involves "breading and frying."(Bad habit—too much frying and too much bread!)

- I have a general dislike toward exercise—I have a "no exercise" habit. (Bad habit—no exercise.)

- A casserole just isn't a casserole without cheese. (Bad habit— foods smothered in cheese. Use nonfat cheese.)

- To me, breakfast is bacon, eggs, and toasted white bread with butter and jelly. (Deadly habit—a bad-for-you breakfast. This is suicide on the installment plan.)

- A meal just doesn't seem complete without dessert—preferably ice cream. (Bad habit—dessert at every meal.)

- My hostess will think I don't like what she fixed if I don't have a second helping. (Bad habit—second helpings.)

- If you put it on your plate you have to eat it. (Bad habit—the "clean your plate" syndrome.)

- If one bite is good, two bites are better! (Bad habit—mindlessly eating more than is necessary.)

- A spoonful of sugar makes everything go down better, not just the proverbial medicine. (Bad habit—sugar consumption.)

- Fried chicken, mashed potatoes, and cream-based gravy is the ultimate comfort food. (Bad habit—equating food with "comfort." How fast do you want heart disease?)

- What's a Saturday night without pizza? (Bad habit—pizza.)

- I can't imagine a hamburger without fries and a cola. (Bad habit—fried foods, sugar drinks, and bread.)

The Top Five Bad Eating Habits I Need to Change

1.

2.

3.

4.

5.

Next to each of these statements, write in bold, large letters: "I WILL CHANGE THIS!"

Bad Excuses

We all tend to use excuses when it comes to fat. Obese people tend to be masters at self-justification. Below are some of the many excuses I've heard through the years for a failure to pursue or maintain fat loss.

EXCUSES FOR NOT LOSING FAT

- My spouse will become jealous if I lose weight and become more physically attractive.

- People will think I'm ill if I lose too much weight.

- If I lose weight, I'll have more wrinkles.

- Eating is my greatest pleasure; take away food and I won't have much joy in life.

- My life is too stressful right now to diet—I can't add one more concern to my life, much less my body fat.

- It will take forever to lose all the weight I should lose and I just can't see myself maintaining a program that long.
- I don't like to cook and plan menus and that's what dieting is all about.
- My work forces me to eat out a lot and I can't imagine losing weight while eating in restaurants all the time.
- My friends would never put up with a special diet.
- I'm not good at making changes.
- When I'm fat I don't have to deal with advances from the opposite sex.
- I'll do it next month.

My Top Three Excuses for Not Losing Fat —Starting Today

1.

2.

3.

Now take your pen and draw a line through each of these statements. Write in the margin to the right of each statement, in large bold letters: "AN EXCUSE I REFUSE TO LIVE WITH!"

Fat Fact

One out of every three Americans is at least 20 percent overweight and about three out of four Americans are heavier than their optimal weight.

REACHING A DECISION

Choosing to lose fat is a personal choice that reflects to a great extent what you choose to believe about yourself. See yourself as a person who can say "YES!" to each of the statements below. Write "YES!" next to each one.

AN I-CAN-DO-IT DECISION

- I do have enough self-discipline to lose fat.

- It's completely acceptable to do this solely for myself and because I want to lose fat.

- I will make the changes necessary in the way I eat and drink.

- I will make the changes necessary in the way I exercise.

- I will learn what is good for my body and then do those things.

- I will see myself as a winner with a positive attitude.

- I will choose to envision myself as a person who has accomplished the goal of fat loss.

- I will make changes in my daily routine and schedule for the betterment of my health.

- I will choose to turn off all negative comments around me that might influence me to stop a fat-loss program.

- I will choose to turn off as many "food cues" as possible—including turning off TV commercials and looking away from food billboards before their messages penetrate my mind.

- I will choose to associate with people who will support and not hinder my pursuit of maximum fat loss.

- I will accomplish a long-term goal and maintain a new pattern of eating and exercising the rest of my life.

- I will have the courage necessary to face any fears I may have about fat loss.

- I will have the fortitude to persevere in my fat-loss program until I reach my goal.

- I will become my physical best.

And here's my signature to attest to the fact that *all* of me believes *all* of the above!

Signature:_____

Date: _____

QUESTION TO CONSIDER
What do you consider to be "too fat"?

DEVELOPING A PERSONAL REASON
FOR LOSING FAT

Deep down inside, you need to have a driving reason for *why* you want to lose fat. It's not enough to make a decision to lose fat. Losing fat must become a deeply held desire of your heart.

A desire has an emotional component to it that compels changes in attitude and behavior. When you truly desire to lose your excess fat, you'll start doing what is necessary. Below are some samples of motivating desires.

REASONS UNDERLYING DESIRE

- to feel and look better in my clothes

- to be in better health

- to have more energy

- to prevent health problems in old age

- to improve my social life

- to cultivate a deep inner conviction that this is the right thing to do

- to have success in this area of my life where I've had little to no success—I'm tired of making resolutions I never keep

- to lower the general pain level and degree of stiffness I feel

- to reduce or eliminate some of the medications I have been prescribed (including lessening my dependence upon antacids, laxatives, and painkillers)

- to spend my health-related dollars more wisely

- to live longer and with greater quality of life

- to feel more like engaging in physical activities and sports that I enjoy

Why have you reached the decision to lose your excess fat? What is your number one reason for wanting to lose fat? What is at the core of your desire to be lean at last, with a leanness that is lasting? Write below in the space labeled "Number One Reason" the primary reason on which your desire is based. If you have more than one reason, list those reasons in the area labeled "Secondary Reasons." You can list as many secondary reasons as you wish. (The more secondary reasons you can cite, the greater your desire is likely to grow.)

My Number One Reason for Losing Fat
(My Heart's Desire)

_____

_____

🥞 Fat Fact

Overweight people have far more joint, ligament, back, and knee problems than slender people.

Secondary Reasons for Losing Fat
(My Heart's Desire)

_____

_____

_____

_____

_____

_____

_____

_____

_____

_____

_____

ACTION STEPS FOR WEEK #1

- Do *not* eat pizza.

- Begin to drink more water—lots more water!

- Do not eat white bread or junk cereals.

- Read *Maximum Fat Loss*.

(I also suggest you order the *Eat, Drink, and Be Healthy* program from my office: 1-800-726-1834.)

QUESTION TO CONSIDER
What can you do to shield yourself against the onslaught of cynicism and negativity that seems pervasive in our society–including the cynicism and negativity that are related to diets, fat-loss programs, good nutrition, and vitamins and other nutritional supplements?

JUMP-START EACH DAY MENTALLY AND PHYSICALLY

Take a few minutes at the start of each day also to recharge your resolve concerning your fat-loss program. I suggest that just before you drink that first morning protein drink or eat breakfast that you sit down in a comfortable chair and spend three minutes just relaxing your body. Concentrate on a complete slackening of the muscles of your legs, pelvis, abdomen, arms, shoulders, and neck—in that order. Think through some of the positive statements that you have written down or established as goals or motivational triggers to help you stay on a fat-loss program.

Close your eyes and visualize yourself as having an abundance of physical energy, being lean and fit and healthy, and having good mental and emotional vitality for doing all that lies ahead for you.

Does this sound too simplistic for you? Try it for a week and I think you'll be amazed at what this three minutes in a morning can do to build new mental habits to go along with your fat-loss program.

REALISTIC GOALS THAT CHALLENGE AND REWARDS THAT MOTIVATE

WEEK #2

CHALLENGE AND CHANGE FOR WEEK #2
Set realistic goals and motivating rewards.

FAT-LOSS TIP

For up to two hours after intense exercise, the body works to restore glycogen directly to the muscles, bypassing the liver and other storage sites, including fat cells.

Goals are far more than dreams. A dream is a vague whim or hope—often no more than snippets of wishful thinking. A goal is something very specific that is set into a timeframe and that has a method for accomplishing the goal attached to it.

> **Dream or Wish:** "Someday I'd like to be thin again."
> **Goal:** "Within twenty weeks, I am going to lose thirty pounds of fat and gain five pounds of muscle, for a net loss of twenty-five pounds, through eating properly and exercising daily."

Throughout this chapter, you are going to be challenged to set goals for yourself. These goals need to be realistic. They need to take into consideration:

- your height

- your bone structure or body frame

- your age

I encourage you to be ambitious in setting goals for yourself. Set an overall fat-loss goal that challenges you, but that is doable. Set other goals that are truly in keeping with the life you intend to live the rest of your life.

Do not seek to lose more than two pounds of fat a week. If you are willing to work out every day, and to do so with a good degree of intensity and diligence, you are likely to gain as much as a pound of muscle a month. That's going to be a net loss of seven pounds a month. A two-pound-a-week fat-loss goal is realistic, doable, and a good goal for most people.

To lose fat at a rate of two pounds a week, you are going to need to reduce your intake of or burn an extra 7000 calories per week.

WHAT IS YOUR BODY FRAME?

To determine your frame size, bend your forearm upward at a ninety-degree angle. Keep your fingers straight and turn the inside of your wrist toward your body. Place your thumb and index finger of your other hand on the two prominent bones on either side of your elbow. Measure this space between your fingers (on your elbow) with a ruler or tape measure. Compare the space with the tables below listing medium-framed men and women. Measurements less than those listed indicate a small frame. Measurements higher than those listed indicate a large frame.

Height in 1-inch heels	Elbow Breadth
Women	
4'10"–5'3"	2' 1/4"–2' 1/2"
5'4"–5'11"	2' 3/8"–2' 5/8"
Men	
5'4"–5'7"	2' 5/8"–2' 7/8"
5'8"–5'11"	2' 3/4"–3'
6'0"–6'3"	2' 3/4"–3' 1/8"
6'4" and over	2' 7/8"–3' 1/4"

Source: "1979 Build Study, Society of Actuaries and Association of Life Insurance Medical Directors of America." Copyright © 1983, 1993 Metropolitan Life Insurance Company.

DETERMINE YOUR IDEAL BODY WEIGHT

For most of the people I have counseled through the years, ideal weight is their weight when they graduated from high school (assuming they were not overweight in high school). A high school senior is generally fully developed and active enough to be fit.

For others, ideal weight is the amount they weighed when they married. Most people try to be trim and fit for their wedding and as they start their married life together.

Below are two tables to help you determine your ideal body weight. These tables have been put out by Metropolitan Life. They reflect the general standard adopted by many physicians.

Ideal Body Weight for Men

Height in Feet/Inches	Small Frame	Medium Frame	Large Frame
5' 2"	125–131	128–138	135–148
5' 3"	127–133	130–140	137–151
5' 4"	129–135	132–143	139–155
5' 5"	131–137	134–146	141–159
5' 6"	133–140	137–149	144–163
5' 7"	135–143	140–152	147–167
5' 8"	137–146	143–155	150–171
5' 9"	139–149	146–158	153–175
5' 10"	141–152	149–165	156–179
5' 11"	144–155	155–169	159–183
6' 0"	147–159	159–173	163–187
6' 1"	150–163	162–177	167–192
6' 2"	153–163	166–182	171–197
6' 3"	157–167	170–187	176–202
6' 4"	161–171	171–187	181–207

(These weights are related to ages 25–59.)

Ideal Body Weight for Women

Height in Feet/Inches	Small Frame	Medium Frame	Large Frame
4' 9"	99–108	106–118	115–128
4' 10"	100–110	108–120	117–131
4' 11"	101–112	110–123	119–134
5' 0"	103–115	112–126	122–137
5' 1"	105–118	115–129	125–140
5' 2"	108–121	118–132	128–144
5' 3"	111–124	121–135	131–148
5' 4"	114–127	124–138	134–152
5' 5"	117–130	127–141	137–156
5' 6"	120–133	130–144	140–160
5' 7"	123–136	133–147	143–164
5' 8"	126–139	136–150	146–167
5' 9"	129–142	139–153	149–170
5' 10"	132–145	142–156	152–173

(These weights are related to ages 25–59.)

YOUR BMI NUMBER

Body Mass Index (BMI) is calculated as weight in kilograms divided by the square of the height in meters (kg/m^2). BMI is independent of age or sex although there are certain limitations to its use—BMI may not be the best index for children, pregnant women, or highly muscular individuals such as athletes.

"Normal" for a person is determined by many physicians as comparing a person's ideal body weight and BMI. Those with a BMI of less than 27 are considered in the acceptable range, with a BMI of 20 to 25 being ideal. Mild obesity is defined as those with a body weight of 20 to 40 percent above the ideal body weight and a BMI of between 27 and 29. Moderate obesity is defined as 40 to 100 percent above ideal body weight and a BMI between 30 and 40. Approximately four million Americans currently have BMIs between 35 and 40. Morbid obesity, also called clinically severe obesity, is defined as 100 percent or more above ideal body weight or a BMI above 40.

BODY MASS INDEX FOR MEN AND WOMEN

The column to the far left is Height in Inches
The numbers across the top of the chart are BMI numbers.

	18	19	20	21	22	23	24	25	26	27	28	29	30	31	32	33	34	35	36	37	38	39	40+
58	86	91	96	100	105	110	115	119	124	129	134	138	143	148	153	158	162	167	172	177	181	186	191+
59	89	94	99	104	109	114	119	124	128	133	138	143	148	153	158	163	168	173	178	183	188	193	198+
60	92	97	102	107	112	118	123	128	133	138	143	148	153	158	163	168	173	179	183	188	194	199	204+
61	95	100	106	111	116	122	127	132	137	143	148	153	158	164	169	174	180	186	191	195	201	206	211+
62	98	104	109	115	120	126	131	136	142	147	153	158	164	169	175	180	186	191	197	202	207	213	218+
63	101	107	113	118	124	130	135	141	146	152	158	163	169	175	180	186	191	197	203	208	214	220	225+
64	105	110	116	122	128	134	140	145	151	157	163	169	174	180	186	192	197	204	209	215	221	227	232+
65	108	114	120	126	132	138	144	150	156	162	168	174	180	186	192	198	204	210	216	222	228	234	240+
66	112	118	124	130	136	142	148	155	161	167	173	179	186	192	198	204	210	216	222	228	234	241	247+
67	115	121	127	134	140	146	153	159	166	172	178	185	191	198	204	211	217	223	230	236	242	249	255+
68	118	125	131	138	144	151	158	164	171	177	184	190	197	203	210	216	223	230	236	243	249	256	262+
69	122	128	135	142	149	155	162	169	176	182	189	196	203	209	216	223	232	236	243	250	257	263	270+
70	125	132	139	146	153	160	167	174	181	188	195	202	209	216	223	229	236	243	250	257	264	271	278+
71	129	136	143	150	157	165	172	179	186	193	200	208	215	222	229	236	243	250	257	265	272	279	286+
72	132	140	147	154	162	169	177	184	191	199	206	213	221	228	235	242	250	258	265	272	279	287	294+
73	140	147	154	161	168	176	182	189	197	204	212	219	227	234	242	250	257	265	272	280	287	295	303+
74	147	154	161	167	175	181	187	194	202	210	218	225	233	241	249	256	264	272	280	288	295	303	311+
75	154	16	167	175	181	187	193	200	208	216	224	232	240	247	255	263	271	279	287	295	303	311	319+
76	161	167	174	180	186	192	198	204	213	221	230	238	246	254	262	271	279	287	295	303	312	320	328+

QUESTION TO CONSIDER
Do you make excuses about what you eat or how much you eat?

IDEAL PERCENTAGES OF BODY FAT

Below are ideal body fat percentages adjusted for age and for sex (male/female):

Age	Males	Females
10–30	12–18%	20–26%
31–40	13–19%	21–27%
41–50	14–20%	22–28%
51–60	16–20%	22–30%
61 and older	17–21%	22–31%

CHECK YOUR THYROID

Take your temperature upon awakening in the morning for four mornings in a row. The ideal range is between 97.8 and 98.2 degrees Fahrenheit. If you are a woman in child-bearing years, you will want to make sure you take your temperature for four days *after* a menstrual period has ended; that's the most accurate time in your monthly cycle for this reading. If your morning temperature is less than it was when you started your diet, your thyroid is now less active. When body temperature is reduced, low-calorie diets stop working.

PERSONAL DATA SHEETS

Personal data sheets have been provided on the next several pages for recording your weight, measurement, and blood work numbers.

You may duplicate the charts below as many times as necessary. I suggest you put these sheets in your fat-loss binder under a section labeled *DATA*. These are sheets you will want to update periodically:

- Data Sheet #1 is to be updated weekly.
- Data Sheet #2 should be updated monthly.
- Data Sheet #3 should be updated annually.

PERSONAL DATA SHEET #1

(update weekly)

Date	Weight Loss from Previous Week	Loss from from Start Date	Total Loss

PERSONAL DATA SHEET #2

(update monthly)

Date _____   For Month of_____

Current Numbers	Compared to Start Number	Net Change

BMI: _____ (A body fat caliper is the most accurate way to
    determine body fat levels. These are available from my office.)

Body Fat Percentage: _____

Measurements: _____

Neck: _____

Upper arm: _____

Above the bust/chest: _____

Bust/chest: _____

Midway between bust/chest and waist: _____

Waist: ("Pulled in"): _____

Waist ("Let out"): _____

Abdomen: _____

Hips: _____

Upper thigh: _____

Knee: _____

Calf: _____

Ankle: _____

QUESTION TO CONSIDER

Do you make excuses to yourself about exercise?

Personal Data Sheet #3

(update annually)

Date: _____   For Time Period:_____
Current Numbers   Compared to Previous Numbers
Cholesterol:
Thyroid Function:
Hormone Levels:

TARGETING YOUR HEALTH GOALS

Below are a set of goal statements for you to complete. Indicate which time frame you are adopting for each goal by circling the word "weeks" or "months."

- Lose_____pounds in_____weeks/months.

- Reduce my percentage of body fat to_____percent in _____weeks/months.

- Improve the texture of my skin and hair in weeks/months.

- Have greater physical strength in_____weeks/months.

- Have greater flexibility, agility in_____weeks/months.

- Lower my cholesterol to a normal range by_____weeks/months.

- Lower my blood pressure to a normal range by _____weeks/months

- Reduce or eliminate these medications by_____weeks/months. (check off all that apply):

  blood pressure medications:_____

  diabetic medications:_____

  antacids:_____

laxatives:_____

painkillers:_____

• Improve my overall energy level by_____weeks/months

IDENTIFYING YOUR PERSONAL NONHEALTH-RELATED GOALS

There are many other very good reasons for seeking to lose fat other than health-related goals. Some of them may be social (from "I want to attract a spouse" to "I want to have more energy for going on recreational outings with my friends"). Some may be psychological (from "I want to feel better about myself" to "I want to know that I have it in me to set a goal and reach it.")

List your nonhealth-related goals below:

Personal Nonhealth Goals

_____

_____

_____

_____

_____

_____

_____

_____

_____

_____

QUESTION TO CONSIDER
Is there any limitation you have experienced that you believe is caused by your obesity?

PUTTING YOUR GOALS ON A CALENDAR

One of the best ways to visually master goal-setting is to write your goals onto a calendar log. A very basic three-month log is provided for you below. You can duplicate it as many times as you desire. I suggest you put it, along with the other charts in this chapter, in a section of your log binder labeled *Goals Log*.

Note your weight today. Note your *ideal* weight. The difference is what you hope to lose. Divide that by two to determine the number of weeks it should take you to reach your goal weight if you are diligent in the way you exercise and eat. Count out the weeks from today until the point that you *should* be at your ideal weight. Write your ultimate fat-loss goal on the calendar for that week.

Setting Interim Weight-Loss Goals

Note your weight today. One week from today, pencil in your weight-loss goal. Next week when you weigh yourself on that day, write in what you have actually lost. Subtract two pounds from that number and pencil in the number for the next week, same day of the week.

Do your short-term goal-setting on a "rolling" basis. Keep looking at just two pounds of weight loss a week.

Goals Log

Month:

Week #1 weigh day/date: Goal weight:
Week's weight loss: Total weight loss:
Week #2 weigh day/date: Goal weight:
Week's weight loss: Total weight loss:
Week #3 weigh day/date: Goal weight:
Week's weight loss: Total weight loss:
Week #4 weigh Day/date: Goal weight:
Week's weight loss: Total weight loss:

Month:

Week #1 weigh day/date: Goal weight:
Week's weight loss: Total weight loss:
Week #2 weigh day/date: Goal weight:
Week's weight loss: Total weight loss:
Week #3 weigh day/date: Goal weight::
Week's weight loss: Total weight loss:
Week #4 weigh Day/date: Goal weight:
Week's weight loss: Total weight loss:

Month:

Week #1 weigh day/date: Goal weight:
Week's weight loss: Total weight loss:
Week #2 weigh day/date: Goal weight:
Week's weight loss: Total weight loss:
Week #3 weigh day/date: Goal weight::
Week's weight loss: Total weight loss:
Week #4 weigh Day/date: Goal weight:
Week's weight loss: Total weight loss:

You may want to write your goals in a calendar, which you can also use for writing other goal-related information (such as days of major events, a special birthday, an anniversary celebration, or a vacation).

A calendar such as this is also good for keeping track of the specific ways in which you *reward* yourself. Again, feel free to duplicate this calendar as many times as you desire. Put these sheets in your log binder under a section tab labeled *goals*.

🥞 Fat Fact

According to the American Cancer Society, cancer deaths overall are 33 percent higher for men and 53 higher for women whose weight is 40 percent or more above average.

CALENDAR FOR GOALS AND REWARDS

Month:

MONDAY	TUESDAY	WEDNESDAY	THURSDAY	FRIDAY	SATURDAY	SUNDAY

ESTABLISHING PERSONAL REWARDS

No set of goals is complete without a plan for rewarding yourself—both for your ultimate goal and your incremental sub-goals.

Rewards add *motivation* to any fat-loss plan. Some of the rewards are virtually automatic—such as improved health, more energy, greater flexibility, less pain, higher self-esteem, and increased ambition and sociability. You can expect these things to come as you lose fat, and in many ways, the improvements in your health and appearance are rewarding.

Other rewards should be tangible—things you can see, touch, and experience. Tangible rewards are especially important if you have more than forty pounds to lose. The first few pounds may not be all that noticeable to you or to others. A tangible reward can help you mark your progress and stay on track.

The rewards you establish for yourself should be big enough to create within you an intense desire to reach your goal. If a reward doesn't motivate you toward positive achievement, set a different reward or aim at a higher goal.

If your reward is a vacation to a particular place, something you will wait to buy until you are lean, or anything else that is of a tangible nature, you might want to cut out a picture that is related to your reward and keep it where you can see it often. If you don't want to put it in public view, you can always tape it to a page and place it at the front of your binder log.

Rewards are personal. What is rewarding to you may not be rewarding to another person. In the end, what you choose as a reward is strictly up to you. In the end, it's up to you to motivate yourself toward reaching the goals you set. It is only if your rewards are *personally* gratifying to you that they will be motivating.

Below is a list of rewards that some of my clients have set for themselves. Use these only to trigger your own ideas. Then list your personal rewards, both in the "Ultimate Reward" and "Incremental Rewards" sections.

GRAND REWARDS FOR ULTIMATE GOAL ACHIEVEMENT

- vacation

- cruise

- trip to see friends/family

- piece of jewelry

- season tickets

- major celebration party

- whirlpool spa

- motorcycle

- sports car

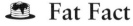 # Fat Fact

As a nation we spend more than $30 billion each year on diet aids and remedies, and that number is rising.

REWARDS FOR INCREMENTAL GOALS ACHIEVEMENT

- manicure or pedicure
- new item of clothing
- weekend away
- new workout equipment
- new exercise outfit/swimsuit
- facial
- massage
- evening at theater, symphony, ballet
- half-day of personal pampering
- piece of exercise equipment for home gym

MY REWARD LIST

Ultimate Reward

_____
_____
_____
_____
_____
_____

Incremental Rewards

_____
_____
_____
_____
_____
_____

MAKE A CONTRACT WITH YOURSELF

A commitment to reach your goals "seals the deal." I recommend that you make a contract with yourself as a statement of your commitment. A sample is provided on the next page, or you can use this as a springboard for constructing your own health-related, goal-reflecting contract.

MY CONTRACT FOR IMPROVING MY HEALTH

I will work to attain a clean (internally and externally), lean body.

I will adopt quality health habits—spiritual, physical, and emotional habits that build genuine wholeness—as the foundation for living quality life.

I deeply desire to make this commitment and I will do all I can to improve my health and accomplish my fat-loss goals:

- I will avoid eating those things that I know are wrong for my body and choose to eat the things that I know are right for good health.

- I will exercise regularly.

- I will drink sufficient water, and take into my body both sufficient fiber and nutrients (including high-quality supplements).

- I will focus on what is good for me rather than give in to what is bad for me.

- I will be grateful for each day's blessings, including the blessing of improving health.

If I do not succeed at the rate I had hoped, I will reexamine what I am doing, make any necessary adjustments, and choose to persevere in my fat-loss program.

If I have a momentary setback at any point, I will consider this a learning experience and I will try again.

I will reward myself for the fat I lose at incremental levels.

I will choose to think well of myself and to see myself as lean and thin someday regardless of what a scale may say or how I may feel emotionally on any given day.

Signed:_____

Date: _____

CHART YOUR PROGRESS

As the months go by, you are going to see real differences in your current chart numbers and the starting numbers you compiled at the beginning of your fat-loss program. Take delight in your own progress!

You may want to chart out your progress on a chart such as the one provided below. Perhaps have one chart for your weight, another for waist measurement, and a third for any other area that you want to watch closely. Feel free to duplicate this chart as many times as you desire, in order to keep track of all the measures of progress you want to monitor.

PROGRESS CHART

Month #1	Month #2	Month #3	Month #4	Month #5	Month #6	Month #7	Month #8

Chart of My _____

ACTION STEPS FOR WEEK #2

- Join a gym to have access to weight-training equipment. (Or you can order my exercise videos: 1-800-726-1834.)

- Make sure you have the right gear for engaging in the exercise program of your choice (for example, jogging, dancing, or walking shoes; swim goggles and earplugs; reflective tape for walking when it is dark). List the items you specifically need to safely and correctly do the aerobic (cardiovascular) exercise of your choice.

• Get a walking partner. (If you can't talk a family member into joining you, call a friend. If none of your friends will join you, join an exercise or walking class.

🥞 Fat Fact

The best thing you can do to prevent diabetes, as well as the best thing you can do to manage it if you already have the disease, is to manage your weight and to lose all excess fat. Never lose sight of the fact that diabetes is a serious disease.

Diabetes:

• is the leading cause of blindness in people age twenty to seventy-four.
• is the leading cause of kidney failure.
• is responsible for as much as 60 percent of the impotency in males over age fifty.
• is responsible severe nerve damage in up to 70 percent of all diabetes.
• is the major cause of stroke in the United States.
• is the leading cause of amputation of lower limbs.
• is known to increase the risk of heart disease by two to four times over normal.

WHEN COMPARING DIET PRODUCTS AND FOODS

Not all "light" or "diet" products are actually low in fat. When comparing products, always make sure you:

- evaluate equal serving sizes
- compare sodium amounts
- compare calories
- compare fat grams
- compare sugar grams

You may find that the low-fat version of a product actually has higher sugar content than the original. You may also find that some so-called "fat-free" products also have as much as .5 gram of fat *per serving*. (That's the legal limit for an item to be labeled fat-free.)

A WORKABLE SCHEDULE AND PLAN

CHALLENGE AND CHANGE FOR WEEK #3
Eat six meals a day, with a calorie total not exceeding ten times
your ideal weight.

FAT-LOSS TIP

Make a deal with a friend! One way to motivate yourself to stay on track with a fat loss program is to make a deal with a friend. If you do not lose two pounds in a given week, pay your friend $10. If he does not lose two pounds, then he pays you $10. Keep this money in a special box or piggy bank. When you reach your goal weight, open your "Bank" and use that money for something that will help you maintain your fat loss . . . perhaps an extended membership at a gym or a piece of equipment for your home gym. Or, if you want, donate the money to your favorite charity.

Calorie Calculations

To determine your calorie total for a day, begin with your ideal weight. Multiply that number by 10 to get your calorie total. For example, you desire to weigh 140 pounds.

$$140 \times 10 = 1,400$$

That's your calorie total for a day. Do not go below this number.

If you currently weigh more than forty pounds over your ideal weight, calculate your ideal weight as thirty pounds less than you presently weigh. That is your calorie total for now. After you have lost ten pounds, readjust your calorie total downward. Do this repeatedly until you are within thirty pounds of your ideal weight. For example, you presently weigh 300 pounds. Your desired weight at the outset should be 270 pounds.

$$270 \times 10 = 2,700$$

When you get down to 290 pounds, recalculate your calorie total. At that time, your desired weight should be 260 pounds (thirty pounds less).

$$260 \times 10 = 2,600 \text{ as a calorie total}$$

Remember—never eat less than ten times your ideal weight in calories!

Question to Consider
Is there someone other than yourself that you are trying to please by losing fat? (Are you really losing fat to please *yourself*?)

Your Daily Calorie Total

your ideal or desired weight:_____
multiplied by ten: _____
Daily Calorie Total: _____

KEEPING A FOOD JOURNAL

A food journal is necessary for you to keep at the outset as you learn how to count calories and determine just how big a healthy meal really is. In keeping a food journal, write down *everything* that goes into your mouth—from breath mint to bite of steak, from one ounce of fruit juice to a bite of zucchini. Be sure to include any sauces, condiments, or salad dressings.

Do *not* fudge on the amount or quantity. If anything, err on the larger side. Consult the calorie counter at the back of this workbook to determine calories per portion.

Do weigh portions of foods when appropriate, especially ounces of meat and dairy products, as well as ounces of fluids.

A place is provided below for you to keep track of your water intake. Do *not* count caffeinated drinks, ice tea, alcohol, fruit juices, or other beverages as part of your water intake even though they may be water-based beverages.

One week's worth of journal sheets is provided for you in this workbook. Feel free to duplicate more pages until you really feel competent at evaluating calories and portion sizes.

🥞 Fat Fact

The proportion of children who are overweight jumped from 5 percent in 1964 to nearly thirteen percent in 1994, the most recent year on record. If that trend has continued, and many believe it has accelerated, one child in three is now either overweight or at risk of becoming overweight.

Food and Water Journal

Date:

Item of Food	Amount/Quantity	Calories

Water Intake:

Time	Ounces

Food and Water Journal

Date:

Item of Food	Amount/Quantity	Calories

Water Intake:

Time	Ounces

Food and Water Journal

Date:

Item of Food	Amount/Quantity	Calories

Water Intake:

Time	Ounces

Food and Water Journal

Date:

Item of Food	Amount/Quantity	Calories

Water Intake:

Time	Ounces

Food and Water Journal

Date:

Item of Food	Amount/Quantity	Calories

Water Intake:

Time	Ounces

Food and Water Journal

Date:

Item of Food	Amount/Quantity	Calories

Water Intake:

Time	Ounces

Food and Water Journal

Date:

Item of Food	Amount/Quantity	Calories

Water Intake:

Time		Ounces

A Check Register for Your Calories

Date: **Starting Calorie Balance:**_____

Food Item   Calories   New Balance

SCHEDULING YOUR MEALS

Below is a sample schedule that provides for six meals in a day, spaced evenly at two-and-a-half-hour intervals. This schedule also identifies the number of calories consumed at each meal. Remember: Your first meal of the day should be the largest, your last meal of the day the smallest. (A large meal can also be consumed after a cardiovascular workout.) If you are doing your cardiovascular workout first thing in the morning, your after-exercise and first meal of the day are one and the same!

Meal	Time	Calories
Breakfast	7:00 A.M. (after aerobics)	375
Midmorning snack	10:30 A.M.	275
Lunch	12:00 P.M.	275
Midafternoon snack	2:30 P.M.	275
Late afternoon snack	5:00 P.M.	275
Evening meal	7:30 P.M.	225
	Total:	1,700 calories

YOUR OWN SCHEDULE

Identify the schedule you intend to keep at the outset of your fat-loss program. Feel free to adjust this after several days to reflect any changes that your schedule may dictate. Try to keep your food intake no more than three and a half hours apart. Ideally, meals should be spaced evenly at two-and-a-half-hour-intervals. As reflected in the example provided, you should make adjustments for those days when you might have an afternoon strength-building (weights) exercise session. If your weight-training workout is coupled with your aerobics workout in the early morning, you might want to add a few more calories to your breakfast meal.

QUESTION TO CONSIDER
What are your first food memories?

Meal	Time of day	Calories
Breakfast		
Midmorning snack		
Lunch		
Midafternoon snack		
Late afternoon		
Evening		

SAMPLE MEALS

Remember that all foods you consume should be chemical, hormone, and pesticide free.

- six egg whites and a small bowl of oatmeal with no- fat milk

- three ounces of skinless chicken and low-glycemic-index vegetables

- three ounces of fish and low-glycemic-index vegetables

- slice of skinless turkey breast with a handful of air-popped popcorn

- one cup of tomato dill soup with an open-faced albacore tuna-salad sandwich on a slice of whole-grain rye bread

- eight ounces of vegetable lasagna, using whole-grain pasta and two ounces of antipasto salad

- one cup of low-salt onion soup and a spinach salad topped with a few slices of red onion and the sections of an orange

- two cups of Chinese vegetables stir-fried with three ounces of chicken

- a three-ounce low-fat turkey burger on one half a whole-wheat bun with slices of tomato, onion, and lettuce

- two cups of whole-wheat pasta primavera and a romaine lettuce salad with nonfat Caesar dressing

- a broiled tomato served with four ounces of broiled fish and a cup of steamed greens (such as chard)

- a two-egg (whole egg or substitute) omelet with two ounces of nonfat cheese or cottage cheese and one and a half cups of mixed tomatoes and chopped green peppers

- two cups of mixed-green salad with nonfat dressing; a half cup of vegetable broth; one and a half cups of steamed broccoli, red peppers, onion, mushrooms, and zucchini topped with two ounces of plain nonfat yogurt; and a half cup of sugar-free applesauce

- a cup of vegetable soup; a lettuce salad topped with sautéed pea pods, mushrooms, and asparagus, and three ounces of lean beef

- a cup of cooked oatmeal topped with a cup of plain, fat-free yogurt and a cup of strawberries

- a spinach salad; a cup of broccoli, peppers, onions, and mushrooms topped by a half cup of marinara sauce; and a half cup of fat-free cottage cheese

- a four-ounce fish fillet, baked or poached; a cup of asparagus; a cup of zucchini; and a mixed salad with nonfat dressing

- two ounces of nonfat cottage cheese topped with several dashes of cinnamon; a half of a grapefruit; and half a toasted whole-wheat bagel (no butter or cream cheese)

- a half a papaya stuffed with a tuna salad made with nonfat plain yogurt, celery, and a few raisins and walnuts

- four ounces of roast lamb with a half cup each of fresh spinach and mushrooms

- eight ounces of nonfat milk, a cup of blueberries, and a cup of whole-grain cereal

- half a whole-wheat pita bread round stuffed with two scrambled eggs, chopped tomato and green pepper pieces, and an apple

- four ounces of turkey breast, one and a half cups of steamed green beans, and a large mixed-green salad and nonfat dressing

- two links of turkey sausage (no nitrate, well-drained), two scrambled eggs, and several slices of tomato and onions

- a cup of vegetarian chili, a slice of whole-grain bread, and a mixed green salad and nonfat dressing

- a cup of plain nonfat yogurt, a quarter cup of wheat germ, and half a grapefruit

- three ounces of chicken breast, a cup of collard greens steamed with onions, and a cup of steamed zucchini

- two eggs scrambled with one ounce of smoked salmon, topped with a little chopped onion and a half teaspoon of capers, and served with a sliced tomato

- twelve ounces of hearty vegetable soup (preferably homemade—watch the sodium content on packaged mixes and canned soups)

- half an avocado with a couple of ounces of Albacore tuna

- half a pear and a half cup of cottage cheese

YOUR OWN MEAL IDEAS

Here's a place to reflect your own creativity—six meals of your own design:

- _____

_____

- _____
  _____

- _____
  _____
  _____

- _____
  _____
  _____

- _____
  _____
  _____

- _____
  _____

PLANNING YOUR DAILY MEALS

Below is a week's worth of forms for planning six meals a day. You should duplicate this chart as many times as necessary. I recommend that you make a binder for these sheets and keep them in a tabbed section labeled *meals*. Planning sheets such as these can be useful in reminding yourself of special meals as you plan your food for the months ahead.

Remember that each meal in the *Maximum Fat Loss* program requires that you have protein, carbohydrates, and fatty acids at each meal. Make sure you are also taking in enough fiber and water.

Fat Fact

Weight loss can occur with loss of water from the body, loss of muscle mass, and loss of vital-organ tissue! *Fat* loss is concerned only with the loss of true *fat*.

DAILY MEAL PLANNING GUIDE

Meal #1
Protein Source:

Carb Source:

Fat:

Fluid:

Fiber:

Meal #2
Protein Source:

Carb Source:

Fat:

Fluid:

Fiber:

Meal #3
Protein Source:

Carb Source:

Fat:

Fluid:

Fiber:

Meal #4
Protein Source:

Carb Source:

Fat:

Fluid:

Fiber:

Meal #5
Protein Source:

Carb Source:

Fat:

Fluid:

Fiber:

Meal #6
Protein Source:

Carb Source:

Fat:

Fluid:

Fiber:

DAILY MEAL PLANNING GUIDE

Meal #1
Protein Source:

Carb Source:

Fat:

Fluid:

Fiber:

Meal #2
Protein Source:

Carb Source:

Fat:

Fluid:

Fiber:

Meal #3
Protein Source:

Carb Source:

Fat:

Fluid:

Fiber:

Meal #4
Protein Source:

Carb Source:

Fat:

Fluid:

Fiber:

Meal #5
Protein Source:

Carb Source:

Fat:

Fluid:

Fiber:

Meal #6
Protein Source:

Carb Source:

Fat:

Fluid:

Fiber:

DAILY MEAL PLANNING GUIDE

Meal #1

Protein Source:

Carb Source:

Fat:

Fluid:

Fiber:

Meal #2

Protein Source:

Carb Source:

Fat:

Fluid:

Fiber:

Meal #3

Protein Source:

Carb Source:

Fat:

Fluid:

Fiber:

Meal #4

Protein Source:

Carb Source:

Fat:

Fluid:

Fiber:

Meal #5

Protein Source:

Carb Source:

Fat:

Fluid:

Fiber:

Meal #6

Protein Source:

Carb Source:

Fat:

Fluid:

Fiber:

DAILY MEAL PLANNING GUIDE

Meal #1

Protein Source:

Carb Source:

Fat:

Fluid:

Fiber:

Meal #2

Protein Source:

Carb Source:

Fat:

Fluid:

Fiber:

Meal #3

Protein Source:

Carb Source:

Fat:

Fluid:

Fiber:

Meal #4

Protein Source:

Carb Source:

Fat:

Fluid:

Fiber:

Meal #5

Protein Source:

Carb Source:

Fat:

Fluid:

Fiber:

Meal #6

Protein Source:

Carb Source:

Fat:

Fluid:

Fiber:

DAILY MEAL PLANNING GUIDE

Meal #1

Protein Source:

Carb Source:

Fat:

Fluid:

Fiber:

Meal #2

Protein Source:

Carb Source:

Fat:

Fluid:

Fiber:

Meal #3

Protein Source:

Carb Source:

Fat:

Fluid:

Fiber:

Meal #4

Protein Source:

Carb Source:

Fat:

Fluid:

Fiber:

Meal #5

Protein Source:

Carb Source:

Fat:

Fluid:

Fiber:

Meal #6

Protein Source:

Carb Source:

Fat:

Fluid:

Fiber:

DAILY MEAL PLANNING GUIDE

Meal #1
Protein Source:

Carb Source:

Fat:

Fluid:

Fiber:

Meal #2
Protein Source:

Carb Source:

Fat:

Fluid:

Fiber:

Meal #3
Protein Source:

Carb Source:

Fat:

Fluid:

Fiber:

Meal #4
Protein Source:

Carb Source:

Fat:

Fluid:

Fiber:

Meal #5
Protein Source:

Carb Source:

Fat:

Fluid:

Fiber:

Meal #6
Protein Source:

Carb Source:

Fat:

Fluid:

Fiber:

DAILY MEAL PLANNING GUIDE

Meal #1
Protein Source:

Carb Source:

Fat:

Fluid:

Fiber:

Meal #2
Protein Source:

Carb Source:

Fat:

Fluid:

Fiber:

Meal #3
Protein Source:

Carb Source:

Fat:

Fluid:

Fiber:

Meal #4
Protein Source:

Carb Source:

Fat:

Fluid:

Fiber:

Meal #5
Protein Source:

Carb Source:

Fat:

Fluid:

Fiber:

Meal #6
Protein Source:

Carb Source:

Fat:

Fluid:

Fiber:

ACTION STEPS FOR WEEK #3

- Eat more vegetables.

- Do not eat processed breakfast cereals.

- Try three new spices or herbs with your foods.

- Stop eating bread in any form. This includes biscuits, pancakes, cornbread and rice cakes.

🥞 Fat Fact

The human body stores and loses fat in the same sequence. When the human body begins to store excess fat, it does so in an orderly way, proceeding from the abdominal area to the deep tissues surrounding the abdomen, followed by the superficial areas around the body, then the buttocks, and lastly, the thighs and arms. When a person begins to lose fat, the order is the same: abdomen first, deep abdominal tissues, superficial areas all over the body, buttocks, thighs and arms.

A KITCHEN INVENTORY

Consider these items as being very helpful tools in your fat loss program:

- Vegetable oil atomizer or lemon-juice spritzer

- A juicer—for making your own fruit and vegetable juices from fresh produce

- A blender—for making protein drinks

- A small accurate scale—for weighing portions of meat and grains

- A grain grinder for preparing your own whole-grain flours

- A steamer or steaming racks—for steaming vegetables and fish

- Food chopper or food processor—for quick chopping of vegetables and fruits

- Plastic containers and bags for storing foods and taking meals to work—taking your own lunches to work is a good way to avoid the temptation of a workplace cafeteria and you'll save money as well!

AN EMPHASIS
ON PROTEIN

CHALLENGE AND CHANGE FOR WEEK #4
Eat sufficient high-quality protein at every meal.

FAT-LOSS TIP

Fill your "spare time" with something other than eating. Sign up for an evening course, do volunteer work, get involved in a social, political, community, or church group! None of those things adds fat to a person's life...rather, you will be expending energy and finding "social" outlets that don't involve cooking and eating.

Your Body's Need for High-Quality Protein

You should be consuming one gram of protein per pound of *lean body mass* per day to provide your body with all the amino acids necessary to support muscle growth and tissue repair. In most cases, about one hundred calories of protein should be eaten at each of your mini meals, or a total of about six hundred calories of protein a day for the average person.

Protein should be the mainstay of your first meal of the day and your last meal of the day. Protein in the evening decreases the muscle-wasting effects that your body experiences overnight. If you are only eating about two hundred calories at your last meal of the day, most of those calories need to be in protein.

When you are losing fat, you need even more protein because your body burns more protein on a low-calorie diet that includes rigorous exercise. You must exercise regularly in order for protein to do its maximum work in your body.

PROTEIN POWDERS

Protein powders are an easy, convenient, and easily measurable means of making sure that you are consuming enough high-quality protein in a day. Make certain the protein you take in contains no hormone, pesticide, or antibiotics influence, and that the product has no artificial sweeteners.

The most common protein products are:

Whey

Whey is found in milk and was originally isolated as a byproduct of cheese production. Whey dissolves well in water, is highly digestible, and has a very good amino-acid profile. It has immunoglobulin proteins that supplement the body's immune system. Make sure you choose a whey protein powder that uses a low-heat, micro-filtration, or ion exchange process in its manufacturing (check the label). The downside is that this type of protein powder tends to be several times more expensive than other protein powders.

Soy Protein

Soy-based protein powders tend to have a concentration of the top five amino acids. Soy protein seems to reduce nitrogen loss and to enhance fat loss during low-calorie dieting. Soy has cholesterol-lowering and triglyceride-lowering effects. It thins the blood slightly and may help in circulation and nutrient delivery of glucose to muscles. It also seems to give the thyroid hormones a boost. This is what my wife and I use.

Egg Protein

Egg protein powders have a good amino-acid profile. They are among the best of the protein powders. I recommend, however, that you save your egg whites to eat as a whole-food source of protein.

Casein

Nonfat cottage cheese is the best source of quality casein protein available. Casein is often an ingredient in other protein powders. It has good digestibility and a high absorption of amino acids, as well as a high glutamine content. It has been shown to increase neurotransmitter activity in the brain and can help with the absorption of amino acids in muscle cells.

Combine your powders.

I recommend that you mix your protein powders for maximum effectiveness, with an emphasis on soy protein powder.

WHOLE-FOOD SOURCES FOR PROTEIN

Chicken

The proverbial chicken breast is still the number one choice of food-source protein. Chicken breast meat is low in fat and high in amino acids. Be sure to take off the skin and grill the meat.

Turkey

Turkey is highly nutritious and lean. Watch out for ground turkey, however—make sure you are getting ground turkey breast, not ground turkey with skin or dark meat. Ground turkey breast has only 1 to 2 percent fat, but turkey with skin or dark meat may have as much as 20 percent fat.

Fish

The fat content of fish varies greatly depending not only on the species of fish but whether they've been packed in oil or water. The fish to avoid are herring, mackerel, pompano, sardines, shad, catfish, shark, and bluefish.

Feel free to indulge in lean fish such as cod, haddock, orange roughy, perch, pike, red snapper, rockfish, sea bass, and albacore tuna. If you are eating canned fish, use water-packed fish.

Eggs

Stick with egg *whites*. Whole eggs do have a high amount of lecithin, which emulsifies the cholesterol in egg yolks, but nonetheless, the real protein power of eggs lies in the white of the egg.

Milk Products

Nonfat milk and fat-free milk products are fine. Anything else should be avoided, even 2 percent, reduced-fat, and other low-fat milks. (Try goat's milk—it is much better for you than cow's milk.)

If the frozen yogurt that tempts you is one gram of fat or less per serving, you may want to treat yourself occasionally. Be aware, however, that most frozen yogurt products have more fat than that and many are sweetened with artificial sweeteners.

Beef

Today's beef products are much lower in fat, calories, and cholesterol than products before 1980. Beef is a great source of protein, B-vitamins, creatine, zinc, and iron. Lean beef is about 72 percent water, 20 percent protein, and only about 7 percent fat. Lean beef is very close to a chicken breast or fish in cholesterol for a three-ounce serving.

Organ Meats

Organ meats (such as liver) are high in protein, but also high in fat and cholesterol. Nuts are also high in protein, but they are also high in fat. I recommend that you stay away from both organ meats and nuts while on a fat-loss program. You may introduce them *occasionally* after you are on a maintenance plan, but never in high quantity or in great frequency.

COMPARING PROTEIN FOODS FOR FAT AND CHOLESTEROL

	Total Fat	Saturated Fat	Cholesterol
Chicken Breast	3.0 grams	0.9 grams	72 mg
Top Round Steak	4.0 grams	1.0 gram	71 mg
Turkey (light/dark)	5.0 grams	1.6 grams	64 mg
Top Sirloin	6.1 grams	2.4 grams	76 mg
Chicken Thigh	9.3 grams	2.6 grams	81 mg

Fat Fact

Losing weight at a rate of two pounds a week allows your body to adjust gradually to the fat loss, without clogging your blood vessels. Be patient! Lose fat slowly and keep it off!

COMPARING CUTS OF BEEF FOR PROTEIN AND FAT

Cut (3-ounce portion)	Calories	Protein Grams	Fat Grams
Brisket	189	27	8
Flank Steak	213	23	9
Lean Ground (10% fat)	169	22	9
T-Bone Steak	182	24	9
Top Sirloin Steak	165	26	6
Rib Eye Steak	191	24	10
Eye Round	143	25	4
Round Tip	157	24	6
Top Round	153	27	4
Shank (Crosscuts)	171	29	5

TED'S SUPER PROTEIN DRINK

This is the protein drink that my wife, my twelve-year-old son, my eighteen-month-old toddler, and I drink daily. All the ingredients are available through my office if you can't find them elsewhere (1-800-726-1834). This is the best nutrient-dense shake recipe I've ever developed. The approximate calorie count is three hundred calories per serving. (We also carry a protein shake "package" through my office.)

Take 1 tablespoon cod liver oil two minutes before drinking your shake (one teaspoon for your children).

(Serving size: three shakes)
1 cup frozen blueberries, or raspberries, or strawberries
2-3 very ripe bananas (peeled and frozen are best)
1 teaspoon natural vanilla extract (optional)
⅛ cup granular lecithin
⅛ cup coarse wheat bran

1 tablespoon powdered vitamin C (may use less until you
    become accustomed to the taste)
¼ scoop ultra glycemix (stops your sweet tooth cravings)
4 scoops pure soy protein
8 ounces crushed ice made from distilled water
8 ounces distilled water (add more as needed)
¼ scoop metagenix multiple vitamin in powdered form

In a large blender, thoroughly mix the above ingredients.
Then add 1 tablespoon Grays Lake kosher gelatin and blend
again.
This shake is delicious.

(Note: Scoop size varies from container to container—each container identified
above has its own scoop.)

ACTION STEPS

- Trim all your meat before eating it. (Trim it once before cooking
  and then a second time before eating!)

- Remove all the skin from poultry before eating it, and ideally
  before cooking it.

- Measure your ounces of protein until you are very sure about
  portion size.

- Eat no bread or pasta or rice—unless you use wild rice.
  (Remember: "bread" includes cakes, pastries, biscuits, pancakes,
  rice cakes, pizza—any product made with flour!)

🥞 Fat Fact

Obesity puts a person at a much higher risk for developing coronary
artery disease, gallbladder disease, high blood pressure, kidney disease,
liver damage, and diabetes.

THE RIGHT KINDS OF CARBS

CHALLENGE AND CHANGE FOR WEEK #5
Eat low-glycemic-index carbohydrates at every meal.

FAT-LOSS TIP

As soon as you recognize you have made a mistake in what you have chosen to eat, how much you have eaten, or the way you have prepared certain foods . . . start anticipating your SUCCESS at the next meal or the next day. Erase the past mistake from your memory bank and consider the next meal to be *the first meal of the rest of your life.*

Low-Glycemic-Index Carbohydrates

Your best sources of carbohydrates on a fat-loss plan are fresh fruits and vegetables that are low on the glycemic index—in other words, fruits and vegetables that are digested slowly and therefore turn to sugar in your bloodstream more slowly. These vegetables and fruits have a low insulin response and they are rich in antioxidants. I go into detail on this topic in my book, *Maximum Fat Loss*.

Eat five portions of low-glycemic vegetables or fruits a day.

Cut out all highly processed carbohydrates—that includes potatoes, white rice, pasta, and bread. In their place, choose wild rice and whole-grain products such as oatmeal and whole-grain Kashi. Definitely leave off the butter and rich sauces that you often use as toppings.

Any high-glycemic grains should be consumed one to two hours *after* a weight-training workout. I don't recommend them at all.

A good balance of carbohydrates to proteins is forty grams of carbohydrate to thirty grams of protein.

FAT-BURNER VEGGIES

These are among the vegetables that are excellent fat-burners and that are low on the glycemic index:

- alfalfa sprouts
- artichoke
- asparagus

- bamboo shoots
- bean sprouts
- bok choy

- broccoli
- brussels sprouts
- cabbage
- cauliflower
- celery
- chard
- cucumbers
- eggplant
- greens (such as beet, collard, dandelion, mustard, turnip)
- lettuce
- okra
- parsley
- pea pods
- peppers (green, red, chilies)
- pickles (dill)
- radishes
- sauerkraut
- soy beans
- spinach
- string beans
- summer squash
- tomatoes
- zucchini

These are also good vegetables to include in your eating plan, although less often:

- beans
- beets
- carrots
- corn
- onions
- peas
- pumpkin
- yellow turnip
- winter squash
- yams

(Some of these vegetables—such as potatoes, eggplant, tomatoes, and bell peppers—need to be avoided if you have arthritis. If you need more information on arthritis call my office.)

QUESTION TO CONSIDER
What makes you feel guilty? (Be specific.)

NEW CHOICES!

We've all heard the phrase "meat and potatoes." On a fat loss program, think "meat and veggies." Name three vegetables you might like to try—perhaps for the first time or perhaps using a new recipe—on your fat-loss program:

1.

2.

3.

GOOD FRUIT CHOICES

Below are fruits, and portion sizes, that are low-glycemic additions to your meals:

- 3 fresh medium apricots
- 1 apple
- 1 banana
- ½ cup blackberries
- ½ cup blueberries
- 1 cup boysenberries
- 1 cup cranberries
- 2 figs
- ½ grapefruit
- 2 kiwifruits
- 2 lemons or limes
- ½ mango
- ½ melon (cantaloupe)
- ¼ melon (casaba, Crenshaw, honeydew)
- 1 nectarine
- 1 orange
- 1 cup papaya
- 1 peach
- 1 pear
- ¼ fresh pineapple
- 2 plums
- ½ cup raspberries
- 1 cup strawberries
- 2 tangerines
- 1 cup watermelon

Many of these can be purchased frozen. Most fruits are excellent to add to a protein shake!

ACTION STEPS FOR WEEK #5

- Do not drink fruit juice. Instead, eat pieces of whole fruit on your fat-loss plan.

- Limit any portion of dried fruits to two ounces. (I recommend that you do not eat dried fruit on your fat-loss plan—its too easy to eat too much at a time. You can add dried fruit in limited quantities to a maintenance program.)

- Eliminate potatoes and bread totally in all forms from your eating plan.

🥞 Fat Fact

Overweight men have a much higher chance of dying of colon, rectal, and prostate cancer than slender men. Overweight women have higher rates of endometrial, gallbladder, cervical, ovarian, and breast cancer than slender women. In breast cancer, overweight women not only have an increased risk of getting the disease, but a greater likelihood of fatality because fat makes it harder to detect tumors early.

EATING *ESSENTIAL* FATTY ACIDS

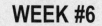

WEEK #6

CHALLENGE AND CHANGE FOR WEEK #6
Eat essential fatty acids at every meal.

FAT-LOSS TIP

A basic rule regarding exercise is this: Exercise the *entire* body. Do something about every muscle group—from the heart muscle to the abdominal muscles, from the lower back, leg, and hip muscles to the upper arm and shoulder muscles. *The areas you don't exercise are the areas where your body will tend to store fat.*

Eat Only the Right Kinds of Fats

There are three basic rules related to your eating of fat:

1. Never eat a fat-free meal.

Some fat needs to be taken along with your protein and carbo-hydrates *at every meal*.

2. Limit your total intake of fat each day.

Be sure to limit your fat intake to about 20 percent of your total daily calories.

3. Eat only the right kinds of fat.

Avoid completely these fats:

- trans-fats (or T-fats)
- polyunsaturated fats or oils
- hydrogenated fats or oils
- partially hydrogenated fats or oils
- hard "shortening" fats (such as Crisco)

Do not use coconut, safflower, or corn oils. Steer clear of all margarine products, including peanut butter made with hydrogenated oil. And stay away from saturated fats—the ones found in meat and dairy products.

QUESTION TO CONSIDER
What emotions have you attached to mealtimes in the past?

OMEGA-3 AND OMEGA-6

The essential fatty acids you need for health and to aid the fat-loss process are Omega-3 and Omega-6 fatty acids. These must be supplied through food—the body cannot manufacture them.

Essential fatty acids are required for the transport and metabolism of both cholesterol and triglycerides. Eating programs with sufficient fatty acids have been shown to lower high cholesterol by as much as 25 percent and high triglyceride levels by up to 65 percent!

Essential fatty acids are also required for the normal development and function of the brain. They are involved in numerous cellular functions—they stimulate metabolism, increase the metabolic rate, increase oxygen uptake, and increase energy production. They also slow the growth of cancer cells. They aid the body by regulating platelet stickiness, arterial muscle tone, inflammatory responses, sodium excretion, and immune functions.

They are critically important to preventing degenerative cardiovascular changes.

FOODS HIGH IN ESSENTIAL FATTY ACIDS

These foods are high in essential fatty acids:

- avocados
- raw nuts and seeds
- olives
- wheat and corn germ

None of these items, however, should become the mainstay of an eating plan. Use them in moderation, no more than twice a week.

Other foods high in essential fatty acids are:

High in ALA: flax oil and walnuts
High in EPA: cod liver oil, cold water fish
High in DHA: algae derived supplements, cod liver oil, and cold water fish

High in GLA: evening primrose oil, borage oil, and black currant seed oil

Fatty Acid Supplements

The easiest way I know to take in all of the essential fatty acids you need each day is to take two two hundred International Units (IU) capsules of cod liver oil and evening primrose oil with each of your meals.

Or you might take one teaspoon of two hundred IU of cod liver oil, and one teaspoon of evening primrose oil (one hundred IU) with each meal.

FAT CONTENT OF COOKED POULTRY

Type	Percent of Calories from Fat	Percent of Fat by Weight
Chicken (Light meat, roasted)		
without skin	23	5
with skin	44	11
Chicken (dark meat, roasted)		
without skin	43	10
with skin	56	16
Turkey (light meat, roasted)		
without skin	19	3
with skin	38	8
Turkey (dark meat, roasted)		
without skin	35	7
with skin	47	12

(Source: *U.S. Department of Agriculture Handbook*, No. 8–5.)

QUESTION TO CONSIDER
What were your favorite childhood foods?

HEALTHY SNACKS

When snacking, reach for something that is nonfat—something that is truly good for your body.

- Munch on celery and carrot sticks.

- Put a scoop of fresh organic applesauce (without any preservatives or added sugar) on top of a scoop of fat-free cottage cheese.

- Eat a small dish of unsweetened Grays Lake kosher gelatin made with natural fruit juice in place of the sugar and water recommended on most gelatin boxes. (Do not use sugar-free gelatin made with aspartame.)

- Have a small slice of watermelon or another piece of fresh fruit.

- Put a few walnuts on a scoop of fat-free yogurt, or enjoy a scoop of fat-free yogurt with a piece of fresh fruit.

- Have a tall glass of herbal iced tea.

- Sip your drink or eat your snack *slowly.* Savor every bite. Give your mind a chance to register a "full" feeling.

Most snack foods are filled with the wrong kinds of fats. Choose fat-free, high-protein snacks!

Identify below three nonfat snack ideas that sound creative and appealing to you:

1.

2.

3.

QUESTION TO CONSIDER
In what ways has being overweight caused you emotional pain?

FIFTEEN SMART-COOKING TIPS

Most people use a significant amount of oil in their cooking. Many foods—not only meats, but also vegetables and cheese—are often breaded and then deep fried. Below are fifteen tips that are easy to incorporate into your cooking routines and which can make a significant difference. Many of them are directly related to the fat content of food.

1. Rather than oil, use very small amounts of nonfat or low-fat flavored vegetable cooking sprays.

2. Use water or a little vegetable or chicken broth rather than sautéing with oil or butter. Vegetable juice and apple cider vinegar can also be used for sautéing. (Watch your pan closely when sautéing with broths and juices.)

3 Use steaming racks for both vegetables and fish. Don't oversteam your foods.

4. Eat vegetables raw whenever possible. Cooking begins the nutritional breakdown of carbohydrates.

5. Drain canned vegetables. Get rid of as much of the sodium as possible. Steam or microwave your canned vegetables rather than boil them—boiling causes more nutrients to be lost.

6. Prepare several portions of chicken or fish at the same time and freeze the unused portions.

7. Always season foods at the table—not as part of the cooking process.

8. Don't taste your cooking unless absolutely necessary. You can consume an amazing number of calories just by tasting a sauce or dish several times.

9. Make a homemade stew, chili, or soup the day before you intend to eat it. Refrigerate the cooked mixture overnight.

That allows you to skim off the fat completely before reheating the dish. The flavors of the ingredients will also have a time to blend thoroughly.

10. Defat your cheese, if you absolutely must use it. Zap an ounce of it in the microwave for two minutes. The fat in the cheese will liquefy and form a pool on top of the cheese. Pour it off. This method works best with mozzarella and cheddar cheeses. Better still—use nonfat cheese.

11. Chop up lettuce and other greens in large batches that can make several salads. Store greens undressed in plastic bags. Use what you need when you need them!

12. Prepare batches of carrots and celery sticks once a week and store them in plastic bags—for quick snacks and for use as part of your meals.

13. Cook enough for two meals. When cooking a meal, cook enough for two or more meals and freeze or store the extra portions for a meal later in the day or week.

14. Use olive oil in making your salads or when you must use oil in cooking.

15. Consider using stevia as a sweetener (never use white sugar or aspartame).

🥞 Fat Fact

If parents are obese, there is more than double the chance that their children will become obese as adults. Genetics plays some role, but the far greater likelihood is that children are imitating their parents' eating and exercise habits. We each tend to eat what our parents taught us to eat, and to exercise in the same way they did.

A NO-FRY VOW

Make a promise to yourself that you will never again fry at least five foods that you routinely fry now. (Sauté is the same as fry when it comes to fat loss!)

1.

2.

3.

4.

5.

ACTION STEPS FOR WEEK #6

Start reading labels on everything you purchase—all canned goods, all packaged items, even vitamin and mineral supplements. Avoid anything that has hydrogenated oils (including partially hydrogenated oil), sugar (including glucose), and high amounts of sodium. Read my book *Maximum Energy* to find out the top ten foods never to eat and why.

Use olive oil or organic butter. Leave all other oils on the grocery shelf!

Do not eat fried foods, and especially do not eat any deep-fried foods (such as french fries).

Take cod liver oil (1 to 2 teaspoons per meal). Be sure to count this oil into your calorie total—cod liver oil has forty-five calories per teaspoon. (The good reasons for cod liver oil are detailed in the *Maximum Fat Loss* book.)

QUESTION TO CONSIDER
Have you used food as a reward, punishment, obligation, or substitute for love?

HAVE YOU TRIED? . . .

Condiments are great for giving a good taste variety to a fat-loss eating plan. Try experimenting with:

- fresh garlic
- allspice
- cinnamon
- cloves
- tumeric
- cayenne pepper
- low-salt, defatted
- broths and onion soup
- saffron
- nutmeg
- powdered mustard
- bay leaves
- fresh salsa
- pumpkin seeds
- walnuts (only a few)
- various types of flavored pepper (key lime, lemon)
- curry powder
- balsamic vinegar
- flavored vinegars
- ginger

PURGING TEMPTATION AND JUNK

WEEK #7

CHALLENGE AND CHANGE FOR WEEK #7
Purge your life of the foods and beverages that are bad for you.

FAT-LOSS TIP

When a snack attack strikes, go to your closet and put on a tight belt, or cinch up your own belt until it is tight. A tight belt can remind you why you are *determined* to lose the excess fat from your body!

PURGING TEMPTATION

What you don't bring home from the grocery store can't make it into the meals you cook at home. What you don't have handy on a nearby shelf or in a kitchen cupboard rarely makes it into your mouth if a craving strikes you. Do your best to preempt snack attacks by purging your pantry and kitchen of foods that you know are high in fat or that are bad for you nutritionally.

TEN THINGS TO DO WHEN A CRAVING STRIKES

Food cravings tend to peak and subside like ocean waves. When a craving strikes, try to wait it out for ten minutes. Most cravings will subside in that amount of time. Don't just sit and wait, however—get up and do something. Distract yourself!

Here are ten things to do instead of giving in to a craving:

1. Take a quick walk, even if its just around the block. (This is not a substitute for a cardiovascular workout. It's a bit of extra exercise to shunt the blood away from your stomach and to put food out of your mind.)

2. Pick up a piece of needlework or handwork or catch up on your mending.

3. Write a note to a friend or head for your computer and send a couple of E-mail messages.

4. Drink a large glass of pure (nonchlorinated and nonflouridated) water. A glass of water is often sufficient to satisfy an empty feeling.

5. Go outside and enjoy the beauty of your garden or the view from your patio or deck. (If your garden isn't beautiful, perhaps pull a few weeds, plant a few flowers, rake a few leaves, or mow a little grass!) Perhaps spend a little time in quiet contemplation or prayer in the beauty of the outdoors.

6. Pick up a book or magazine and immerse yourself in it. Concentrate on what you are reading, not on the food you thought you needed.

7. Take a shower or soak for ten minutes in your whirlpool tub.

8. Surf the Internet.

9. Polish two pieces of furniture in your house (or clean a window, or polish a mirror or two). You might be amazed at how many household chores you can get done in a short five-minute spurt of effort designed to take your mind off a food craving!

10. Call a friend in your support group.

YOUR OWN BATTLING-THE-CRAVINGS STRATEGIES

Name five additional things *you* might do to outlast a craving:

1.

2.

3.

4.

5.

AVOID THE SNACK ATTACK

Prevention is the best offense! Here are specific things you can do to avoid having a snack attack:

Don't skip meals!

This is especially important for breakfast. Skipping a meal signals your body that you are moving into starvation mode and your body will automatically move to reduce your metabolic rate. Those who skip meals tend to "binge" at a future meal. Skipping a meal also impairs your body's ability to recover from exercise.

Eat enough fiber.

Fiber gives a feeling of fullness with less food, and it also improves the stability of blood sugar levels. The body uses more energy—burns up more calories—in absorbing high-fiber foods than low-fiber ones.

Do not chew gum.

It increases the flow of gastric juices that trigger hunger.

Anticipate the timing of when a snack attack is likely to occur.

Some people get into habits of eating specific things at specific times—recognize those habits in your life.

Drink or munch a small amount of a "green food."

Do this about an hour before you usually had a snack food in your old eating pattern. Green foods, such as spirulina, chlorella, and barley green extracts are nutrient-dense and low-calorie super foods. Many contain generous amounts of amino acids along with essential fatty acids, vitamins, and trace minerals. They can energize you without adding empty calories to an eating plan. These foods are available in powdered form, tablets, and capsules.

Don't binge.

A binge can actually stimulate your cravings the second day, and it's almost as if you are back to square one in trying to motivate yourself to maintain a fat-loss program.

Eliminate as many "food cues" as possible.

Food cues are usually visual images that trigger a desire for a specific food. Most of these cues come via television and radio. Try turning off television and the radio for awhile.

Avoid the food court.

When you're at the mall, do your best to avoid all areas where food is offered. The aroma alone can trigger a hunger craving.

Avoid high-glycemic carbohydrates.

They turn to sugar quickly and spike the blood sugar levels in the body. The body then responds by dumping insulin into the bloodstream. This causes storage of the extra sugar as fat. It can also lower the blood-sugar level *too* much, which causes hunger and, specifically, a craving for carbohydrates. The cycle continues. It's the carbohydrate rollercoaster that keeps many people trapped in perpetual dieting and hunger pangs.

Eat six meals a day—each of which is high in protein and which includes low-glycemic carbohydrates (fresh vegetables and fruits low on the glycemic index.) For more information on this topic order my tape series *Forever Fit*.

Your Ideas for Preventing Snack Attacks

Add your own ideas for preventing snack attacks:

1.

2.

3.

GROCERY SHOPPING STRATEGIES

Here are some suggestions for fighting the fat-loss battle at the grocery store:

Shop from a list.

After you have decided what you are going to eat as your basic meals in any given week, make a shopping list. Stick to your list. Don't let your cart wander into aisles that don't have items you need.

Don't shop hungry.

Don't go to the story hungry. Period.

Stay out of bad-for-you aisles.

I suggest you head immediately for the fresh produce section of the store upon arrival, then go to the meats section, and then head for the check-out stand. Stay out of the aisles that feature cereals, processed foods, pasta and bread items, and the general cookie, candy, and sweets aisles.

Consider shopping at a nutrition or health-food market.

Look for organic produce, meats, and milk products.

RESTAURANT TIPS

Here are twenty-five tips for maintaining your fat loss program when "eating out" at restaurants.

1. Choose to eat out less often. You'll face far fewer temptations to binge or to eat the wrong foods.

2. Decide in advance of going to a restaurant what you intend to order. Don't even pick up the menu.

3. Order first. Refuse to be enticed by what others may order.

4. Order foods baked or grilled rather than fried. Especially avoid breaded-and-fried foods.

5. Ask your server not to bring any bread to the table.

6. Ask for steamed vegetables rather than the potato (or rice or pasta) that comes with many meals. (Choose low-glycemic veggies if you are given an option of vegetables.)

7. Dress your salad with a nonfat vinaigrette. If the restaurant doesn't have a no-fat vinaigrette, ask for a little olive oil to be served with several wedges of lemon and ground pepper. Ask for the dressing or these ingredients for a make-your-own dressing to be served to you on the side.

8. Only use salad dressing on every third or fourth bite of salad.

9. Look for low-fat, low-calorie, and heart-healthy items on a menu. Also look for an explanation that tells you how many calories or fat grams these options have. Choose a fish steak over a beef steak.

10. Order everything à la carte. Sometimes soup and salad can be a meal.

11. Order an appetizer as your main course. An appetizer plus a small dinner salad or a small cup of vegetable soup can be a meal in itself!

12. Order any sauces to be served on the side.

13. If cheese is part of the menu item, ask that it be left off.

14. Split a meal. Simply ask for a second plate and do the dividing yourself. Take home half or share the meal with someone else at your table. My wife and I do this all the time.

15. Ask for a "lunch portion." Many menus now have an option of a "lunch size" or "dinner size" entrée.

16. Eat only half of what you are served. At the time you order your meal, ask your waiter for a take-home box. Divide your meal in half even before you take the first bite. Depending on the size of the portions being served at the restaurant, you may be able to take home two meals!

17. Leave some food on your plate. Discipline yourself to leave a few bites of food on your plate. What you don't put into your mouth can't find its way to empty fat cells.

18. Ask for an antipasto or vegetable tray as an appetizer. You'll usually find carrots, celery, and peppers on such a tray. Enjoy! These items are great to add to a green salad.

19. If you're food isn't prepared the way you want it, send it back to the kitchen with specific instructions. Don't be embarrassed to do this. You're the one paying for the food.

20. Ask for fruit or cottage cheese to be substituted on any breakfast platter that features toast or pancakes.

21. Choose clear broth soup rather than cream-based soup.

22. Choose fresh fruit for dessert.

23. Avoid any item that is labeled "deluxe." That usually means its smothered in a fatty sauce or cheese.

24. Avoid ordering casseroles.

25. If you are given an option of restaurants, choose the one that you know has a salad bar so you can make your own selection.

Fat Fact

Only about four hundred grams (sixteen hundred calories) of glucose can be stored in the body at any one time. The liver holds about one hundred grams and the muscles about three hundred grams. Anything above four hundred grams gets stored in *fat cells!*

TIPS FOR SPECIALTY RESTAURANTS

Mexican

Ask for corn tortillas rather than ones made with flour. Choose a chicken taco or tostada made with a baked or steamed tortilla. Check the menu for a vegetarian burrito (and ask for the tortilla to be corn rather than flour).

Italian

Stick to a salad, steamed vegetables, and a broiled fish or chicken entrée.

Chinese

Most Chinese food is very high in fat. Look for stir-fried vegetable dishes and use minimal rice. If you have your option of Oriental restaurants, choose Thai or Vietnamese—the food tends to be lighter with far less oil used in the preparation of most dishes. Never eat at a Chinese restaurant that uses monosodium glutamate (MSG)—this substance has been shown to cause brain damage. Call in advance to see if the restaurant uses MSG.

Steakhouse

Order the leanest steak on the menu. Leave off the loaded baked potato and substitute steamed vegetables and a dinner salad instead.

Greek

Look for chicken shish kebab, a salad *without* feta cheese, anchovies, or olives. Also good is plaki, a fish dish cooked with tomatoes, onions, and garlic.

Breakfast Diner

Order a fruit salad and cottage cheese, or a veggie omelet made with egg whites only.

WHEN GOING TO A PARTY . . .

Pass on the potato chips, tortilla chips, and pretzels. Avoid that end of the buffet table.

Instead of "two scoops" . . . serve yourself only one small spoonful or scoop.

If the party is a potluck, choose to bring a vegetable platter with a nonfat-yogurt-and-fresh-dill dip. Stick mainly to what you bring to the party!

Stay away from the open bar. Ask for a glass of water with lemon or lime wedges.

Limit yourself to one serving along the buffet table (or at the dining table).

Fill your plate with veggies and leave off the dip.

Take along a small toothbrush in your purse or pocket. Excuse yourself to the bathroom and brush your teeth after you know you've had your calorie limit. You'll be less apt to reach for another bite after you've brushed your teeth.

ORDER A SPECIAL MEAL

If you are traveling by air, call the airline twenty-four hours before take-off to order a special meal. Ask for pure-vegetarian and no-oil meals or a fruit plate. You can always put some fresh-vegetable snacks in a baggie and carry them on board with you in your purse or your carry-on luggage.

EATING OUT AT FAST-FOOD SPOTS

If you can't avoid eating out at a fast-food restaurant, here are some tips to "defat" the experience:

- Choose one item and eat it slowly.

- Choose grilled or roasted chicken—no breading, no deep-fat frying. Grilled chicken is great on a salad with nonfat vinaigrette dressing.

- Ask for any "special sauce" to be held. The same for all mayonnaise or cheese.

- Ask for extra lettuce and tomatoes.

- Use mustard or a fat-free dressing as a condiment rather than ketchup (which can have lots of sugar).

- Spice up your chicken with mild or hot sauce (salsa or pico de gallo) or jalapeños.

- Add pickles for extra taste.

- If side orders are available at a deli, look for steamed vegetables or fruit salad.

- Make sure all the skin has been removed from chicken or turkey items. If you have your choice between white and dark meat, choose white.

- If you're at a fish place, make sure the fish is baked, not breaded or fried.

Just about any food item from a fast-food place can be helped by adding a little vinegar and black pepper!

QUESTION TO CONSIDER
Are all of your emotional and spiritual needs being met? If not, what can you do to meet those needs apart from eating?

EXPERIMENT!

Most Americans are uncreative when it comes to food choices. Try some new vegetables or fruits from the fresh-produce section. Try some new recipes from a low-fat or nonfat cookbook. (My wife has an excellent one—you can order it from our office: 1-800-726-1834.)

If you don't know how to prepare a fruit or vegetable, ask the person who works in the produce section. If that person doesn't know, ask to talk to the manager of the produce section.

Take a moment to list three new foods you've always wondered about and decide that you are going to try them as part of your fat-loss program:

1.

2.

3.

🥞 Fat Fact

At any given time, from one quarter to one half of all adult Americans are on some sort of diet.

AT THE TABLE

Here are some tips for your at-home meals:

- Consider using small plates for your meals. A full bread-and-butter plate or salad plate is likely to be perceived by your mind as a full plate of food.

- Pay close attention to every bite you put into your mouth.

- Serve your plate in the kitchen directly from the cooking pans and don't go back for second helpings!

- Drink a large glass water even before you take your first bite of a meal.

- Eat slowly. Thoroughly chew your food—a good trick for slowing your eating is to set your food down between each bite or to put down your fork between each bite and not pick it up again until you have thoroughly chewed and swallowed what is in your mouth and followed it with a sip of water.

- Even if you are eating alone, sit down at a dinner table to eat. Don't mindlessly munch away while watching television.

What additional ideas can you come up with for changing the way you eat a meal with your family, friends, or by yourself? List three:

1.

2.

3.

QUESTION TO CONSIDER
What words come to your mind when you hear the word *exercise*?

PANTRY-PURGING CHECKLIST

Remove from your pantry, kitchen cupboards and shelves all of the following:

- peanut butter
- any item that has a long list of preservatives
- margarine
- Crisco or other shortening
- all products that contain aspartame (NutraSweet)
- all products that have sugar as the first ingredient on the label
- all products that have hydrogenated or partially hydrogenated fats

- all white flour

- all white rice

- all bread and pasta products that are not whole-grain

- all processed cereals that are not whole-grain

- all aspartame sweetened products

(My *Eat, Drink, and Be Healthy* tape series give details in this area: 1-800-726-1834)

ACTION STEPS FOR WEEK #6

- Purge your pantry and kitchen cupboards and shelves *this week!*

- Eliminate white rice from your eating plan. (Eat only small portions of wild rice.)

- Eliminate regular pasta from your eating plan. (Later, after you have reached your fat-loss goal, you may add whole-grain pasta to your eating program in limited quantities and only occasionally.)

Fat Fact

One out of every four teenagers presently carries enough excess weight to put him or her at high risk of heart attack, stroke, cancer, gout, and other serious health problems later in life . . . and that's regardless of whether the individual slims down as an adult.

FLUSHING THE TOXINS FROM YOUR BODY

WEEK #8

CHALLENGE AND CHANGE FOR WEEK #8
Drink half your weight in ounces of pure water every day.

FAT-LOSS TIP

Rather than focus on one meal that wasn't healthy, focus on the meals that were good ones. Say to yourself, *Today was an eighty-percent successful today. Tomorrow I'm going for a hundred percent.*

YOUR NEED FOR PURE WATER

Your body *needs* water. It is not an optional element. For your body to function properly, and especially for all of the metabolic processes related to fat loss to work as they were created to work, you *must* drink sufficient water every day.

Drink pure distilled water. If you don't have a water purifier, purchase one. (Call my office if you need advice about this.) Make sure the purifier uses a reverse-osmosis or steam-distillation process.

Many people think they drink more water than they do. I recently heard about a young man who thought he was drinking a gallon of water a day. He decided that for every glass of water he drank, he'd pour an equal size glass into an empty gallon milk jug he brought to his work place. At the end of the day he was shocked to discover the gallon container was only about a third filled. From then on, he filled that gallon jug first thing in the morning from the pure-water source his employers had provided and he made sure that by lunch time he had emptied half of the container, and the remaining half by the time he went home at six o'clock in the evening.

Carry a water container with you. Keep the fluids flowing all day. If you are at home, fill a gallon container with pure water and place it in the refrigerator. Pour a large glass (twelve to sixteen ounces) out of the container before each of your meals. Try to drink this glass five to ten minutes before you eat. Avoid drinking with meals. Keep a log, if necessary, to make certain that you drink enough water in a day.

You should be drinking half of your weight in ounces every day. In other words, if you weigh 240 pounds, you should be drinking 120 ounces of water a day. That's fifteen eight-ounce glasses. If you weigh 160 pounds, you should be drinking 80 ounces a day. That's ten eight-ounce glasses.

It's okay to drink *more* than this amount. Just don't drink less.

When making ice, be sure to use distilled water.

Are you concerned about being in the bathroom all day? You won't be. But you probably will be there more often. That's good. Along with the water you are eliminating, you are eliminating toxins and fat globules from your body!

🥞 Fat Fact

Overweight people statistically suffer from more colds and infections than lean people.

WATER-BASED BEVERAGES AREN'T THE SAME AS WATER

Water-based beverages, such as coffee and tea, aren't the same as drinking water. In fact, for every cup of coffee or tea you drink, you should be drinking an *extra* glass of water. Caffeine is a diuretic and should never be used on a fat-loss program.

Be cautious in your use of sparkling water products. They often have a high sodium content and actually lower blood oxygen levels.

Also be extremely cautious in your use of "flavored" waters. They are usually high in sugar. The same goes for juice drinks—they often have very little juice and are mostly sugar.

Say no to alcohol.

Alcohol not only adds extra calories to your eating plan, it decreases your body's ability to burn fat.

Say no to diet sodas.

And finally, say no to diet drinks. Most of them are made with aspartame, which lowers brain seratonin levels. This in turn causes carbohydrate cravings. By eating more carbohydrates, you *gain* body fat—its ironic, but drinks that are supposed to help you lose weight may actually cause you to gain more weight! Aspartame, often listed or purchased as NutraSweet or Equal, also has been linked to numerous brain and other physical disorders—all of which are negative and some of which are life-threatening. (Please read the *Maximum Fat Loss* book for more information about aspartame and a list of other side effects associated with aspartame.)

AVOID ALL ASPARTAME DIET PRODUCTS

Aspartame, usually marketed under the name NutraSweet, is used in more than nine thousand products on the market today. Avoid them all! Look for aspartame in these common items:

- instant breakfast drinks
- gelatin
- breath mints
- tabletop sweeteners
- sugar-free chewing gum
- instant teas and coffees
- cocoa mixes
- frozen desserts
- flavored coffee and tea
- beverages
- puddings
- gelatin desserts
- juice beverages
- soft drinks
- laxatives
- some multivitamins
- milk drinks
- sugar-free yogurt
- some pharmaceuticals
- wine coolers
- topping mixes
- breakfast cereals

 Fat Fact

Excess fat is the culprit associated with health problems, not necessarily excess weight. It is the percentage of fat in your body, not the overall weight number you see on the scale, that should be your primary concern.

ACTION STEPS FOR WEEK #8

- Say no to caffeine—in all forms! That includes caffeinated tea, chocolate drinks, cocoa, and cola soft drinks and other drinks that are spiked with caffeine.

- Say no to alcohol—in all forms! That includes wine, beer, liquor, liqueur extracts, mixed cocktails, alcohol-laced coffees, and wine coolers.

- Say no to diet drinks and all other products sweetened with aspartame (NutraSweet or Equal).

QUESTION TO CONSIDER

What can you do to shield yourself against the onslaught of cynicism and negativity that seems pervasive in our society—including the cynicism and negativity that are related to diets, fat-loss programs, good nutrition, and vitamins and other nutritional supplements?

TRANSPORTING THE FAT OUT OF YOUR BODY

WEEK #9

CHALLENGE AND CHANGE FOR WEEK #9
Take in sufficient fiber every day.

FAT-LOSS TIP

Make your meals "beautiful." Appearances DO count. Set a pretty table for some of your meals. Use your best china, silver, and linens. Make "thin" something worth celebrating!

THE BASICS ABOUT FIBER INTAKE

Most Americans do not get enough dietary fiber in a day. Your system needs adequate fiber for two main reasons:

1. Soluble fiber attaches itself to blood fats and creates a complex that removes these fats from the blood system. The net result is an elimination of fat from the bloodstream.

2. Insoluble fiber forms a bulk mass that sweeps bodily wastes, fatty globules, and toxins from the intestinal track and colon.

Dietary fiber has been shown to help lower cholesterol, lower blood pressure, and reduce atherosclerosis (hardening of the arteries), as well as to help with hemorrhoids. High-fiber diets are especially helpful to diabetics with Type II diabetes.

Amount Per Day

You should be eating between twenty-five and thirty grams of fiber a day. In order to take in this much fiber, you must eat at least five servings of fresh fruits and vegetables daily. You should *always* have fiber as part of your breakfast meal. This is why I include it with my protein shake.

GOOD SOURCES OF FIBER

Good sources for fiber include:

- whole, fresh vegetables and fruits, including their skin
- bran—the outer husk of most grains (Look for whole bran or whole-grain products.)

- psyllium husks—a fiber supplement that should be taken before a meal with a large glass of water. (The dosage is usually one tablespoon of psyllium husk powder.) I do not recommend that you use psyllium every day. Do not exceed recommended dosages; too much psyllium can strip the acidophilus—helpful bacteria—from your colon.

- glucomannan—a fiber supplement that is derived from the edible root of the konjac plant. (This product is available in capsules or tablets, as well as in wafer and candy form. The recommended amount is one thousand milligrams. It should be taken with eight ounces of water a half hour before a meal.)

When taking fiber supplements, start out with less than the recommended dosage and let your system adjust to the added fiber over a two- or three-day period. Chew any fiber wafer supplements very slowly and be sure to take them with water.

🥞 Fat Fact

Once a person passes the physical age of twenty, he or she loses 6 to 7 percent of their total muscle mass *every ten years* unless that person does strength-building exercise (also called *resistance* or *weight-training* exercise) on a regular basis.

DO THE MATH

Take a look at the Gram Counter at the back of this workbook. The last column on the right is fiber grams. Scan through the list and note those foods that are high in fiber. List below five foods that you enjoy and that are high in fiber and make a promise to yourself that you will incorporate them into your eating plan.

(Note as you scan the Gram Counter how difficult it is to get enough fiber in a daily diet. I hope this will underscore for you the importance of taking fiber supplements.)

HIGH-FIBER FOODS TO INCLUDE IN MY EATING PLAN

1.

2.

3.

4.

5.

QUESTION TO CONSIDER
Is there something you'd really like to do but don't think you *can* do as long as you are obese?

ACTION STEPS FOR WEEK #9

- Limit your salt intake.
- Stop drinking or eating whole-milk products—only drink or eat no-fat milk, yogurt, cottage cheese, and cheese.
- Start taking supplemental fiber every day.
- Remember to take cod liver oil with each meal.

Fat Fact
Overweight people have far more joint, ligament, back, and knee problems than slender people.

AEROBICS: SETTING THE TONE AND TEMPO FOR EACH DAY

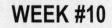

WEEK #10

CHALLENGE AND CHANGE FOR WEEK #10
Do cardiovascular (aerobic) exercise five times a week for twenty-five minutes in the morning before eating anything.

FAT-LOSS TIP

Make a list of things of three things that you intend to do once you have lost weight. (Target those things that you don't think you can do, or which you don't feel like doing.)

THE BENEFITS OF EXERCISE

The major benefits of exercise are:

- Exercise increases lean body muscle mass.

- Strength-building exercise (also called weight training) *is the only way to reshape your genetically predisposed body type.*

- Exercise burns fat.

- Exercise raises a person's metabolic rate.

- Exercise increases the sensitivity of cells to insulin, which allows the pancreas to produce less insulin and not become over taxed.

- Exercise causes the brain to release endorphin neuropeptides, which have been shown to have beneficial effects on the immune system.

- Exercise also reduces the level of stress hormones, particularly the catecholamines. When the body has too high a level of stress hormones, immunity suffers.

QUESTION TO CONSIDER
When you see overweight people, what do you think about them?

THE THREE MAIN TYPES OF EXERCISE EVERY PERSON MUST DO

If you are truly serious about maximum fat loss, you need to include three types of exercise in your weekly routine:

1. cardiovascular exercise (aerobics)

2. strength-building exercise (weights; also called resistance exercise)

3. flexibility exercise (stretching)

Even if you haven't exercised regularly for years, you should start doing all three kinds of exercise. Here's how to get started:

l. If you haven't exercised regularly in awhile, see your physician. Make sure you do not have any cardiovascular problems that might limit your exercise.

2. Set modest goals for yourself as you begin. Don't be reluctant to start out at a very simple, easy level.

3. Make certain that you have adequate "gear" for the type of exercise you intend to do. If you plan to walk as your cardiovascular exercise—which I recommend—make sure you have good walking shoes that give adequate support and cushioning to your feet.

4. Adequately warm up. Don't head out walking, cycling, or even swimming at full speed. Walk, cycle, or swim slowly for a few minutes to warm up your muscles, and then increase your speed for the bulk of your exercise time. Walk slowly for the last few minutes of your exercise session to give your muscles an opportunity to cool down.

I have exercise videos for people at all levels of ability. You can call my office.

CARDIOVASCULAR EXERCISE

You should be doing some kind of continuous cardiovascular exercise for twenty to thirty minutes at least three and preferably five times a week. Cardiovascular exercise is also called aerobics exercise.

Cardiovascular exercise is aimed primarily at the health of the heart, lungs, and the complex network of blood vessels in your body (arteries, veins, and capillaries). Blood vessels and the heart are just like your muscles—they grow stronger with regular use and healthy exercise. The goal of cardiovascular exercise is to accelerate the heart rate for a sustained period of time and to burn body fat if needed.

If possible, engage in cardiovascular exercise first thing in the morning before any calories are eaten or drunk. (Water is okay to drink before cardiovascular exercise.) Exercising on an empty stomach causes the body to release glucagon from the pancreas to facilitate the burning of existing fat deposits for fuel.

I recommend *walking* as the best cardiovascular exercise for overfat people and people over forty. It's much easier on the ligaments of the knees and hips. I also highly recommend the Precor EFX544 eliptical runner—this is what my wife and I use in our daily workouts.

Other than walking, the most popular cardiovascular exercises for the overfat are swimming, cycling, and low-impact aerobics.

Don't try to accomplish your ultimate cardiovascular exercise goals the first day out! Bear in mind that you didn't get out of shape in a day and you aren't going to get back to a level of fitness in a day. If you can't walk fast enough at the outset to get your heart to a true cardiovascular work-out rate, walk twenty minutes at the pace you *can* walk. Stay with your program and you will improve.

KEEP A LOG

Keep a log of your cardiovascular workouts. Record the date, length of your exercise period, and the distance you cover. Also note any pain or discomfort you feel when exercising. Note, too, any emotional feelings you had while walking—such as a heightened awareness of your surroundings, a greater appreciation for nature, a new feeling of energy, a new awareness of the movement of your body.

You will also want to record your flexibility and strength-building exercises. On the back side of each cardiovascular log sheet, you will find a place to record your flexibility and strength-building workouts. More information is provided about how to complete the flexibility and strength-building logs in the next chapter.

Log sheets for one month are provided in this workbook. I encourage you to duplicate these sheets and to maintain an ongoing log. These log sheets cover five cardiovascular workouts a week, and four flexibility and strength-building workouts a week.

Fat Fact

Fat women are less fertile than thin women and have twice the likelihood of giving birth to babies with spina bifida. Complications of pregnancy are far more common in overweight women than in thin women.

STAY AWAY FROM DIET PILLS!

The only product currently approved by the U.S. Food and Drug Administration (FDA) for weight-loss purposes is phenylpropanolamine (PPA). You'll find it in Dexatrim and Acutrim, as well as in some cold medications such as Contact and Dristan. It's actually an ingredient in more than a hundred medications. Americans annually take sixteen billion doses of PPA, four billion of which are in the form of diet pills. Chemically, the structure of PPA is very similar to amphetamines.

Since the 1980s, numerous scientific and medical studies have questioned the effectiveness of PPA. Most have found that actual weight-loss effects are meager. These studies *have* found, however, that PPA can cause blood pressure problems when combined with caffeine. I do *not* recommend that you take PPA. It has also been linked to strokes. There are numerous nutritional supplements that can help curb appetite—supplements that *work*, which have no side effects, and which are healthful in other ways besides appetite curbing.

If you are considering any diet pill or product, read the label very closely. Take heed to any warnings or precautions. These pills are potent. If there are potential side effects, believe what the label says. Never exceed the recommended dosage. In fact, if you *must* take one of these products, take far less than the recommended dose to see how your body handles the chemicals. If you find your sleep disrupted, or if you experience tremors, nervousness, heart palpitations, or tingling sensations, stop taking the product immediately.

Virtually *all* diet pills or products are not considered safe for pregnant or lactating women, people under the age of eighteen, and those with high blood pressure, epilepsy, glaucoma, thyroid disease, or heart disease.

Exercise Log Sheet for the Month of:
Cardiovascular Exercise

Date	Length of Workout	Distance Covered	Physical Notes	Other Notes

Strength-Building and Flexibility Exercise Sessions

Date	Exercise Set Performed	Repetitions/ Weight	Physical Notes

Exercise Log Sheet for the Month of:
Cardiovascular Exercise

Date	Length of Workout	Distance Covered	Physical Notes	Other Notes

Strength-Building and Flexibility Exercise Sessions

Date	Exercise Set Performed	Repetitions/ Weight	Physical Notes

Exercise Log Sheet for the Month of:
Cardiovascular Exercise

Date	Length of Workout	Distance Covered	Physical Notes	Other Notes

Strength-Building and Flexibility Exercise Sessions

Date	Exercise Set Performed	Repetitions/ Weight	Physical Notes

Exercise Log Sheet for the Month of:
Cardiovascular Exercise

Date	Length of Workout	Distance Covered	Physical Notes	Other Notes

Strength-Building and Flexibility Exercise Sessions

Date	Exercise Set Performed	Repetitions/ Weight	Physical Notes

Exercise Log Sheet for the Month of:
Cardiovascular Exercise

Date	Length of Workout	Distance Covered	Physical Notes	Other Notes

Strength-Building and Flexibility Exercise Sessions

Date	Exercise Set Performed	Repetitions/ Weight	Physical Notes

Exercise Log Sheet for the Month of:
Cardiovascular Exercise

Date	Length of Workout	Distance Covered	Physical Notes	Other Notes

Strength-Building and Flexibility Exercise Sessions

Date	Exercise Set Performed	Repetitions/ Weight	Physical Notes

Exercise Log Sheet for the Month of:
Cardiovascular Exercise

Date	Length of Workout	Distance Covered	Physical Notes	Other Notes

Strength-Building and Flexibility Exercise Sessions

Date	Exercise Set Performed	Repetitions/ Weight	Physical Notes

Exercise Log Sheet for the Month of:
Cardiovascular Exercise

Date	Length of Workout	Distance Covered	Physical Notes	Other Notes

Strength-Building and Flexibility Exercise Sessions

Date	Exercise Set Performed	Repetitions/ Weight	Physical Notes

Exercise Log Sheet for the Month of:
Cardiovascular Exercise

Date	Length of Workout	Distance Covered	Physical Notes	Other Notes

Strength-Building and Flexibility Exercise Sessions

Date	Exercise Set Performed	Repetitions/ Weight	Physical Notes

Exercise Log Sheet for the Month of:
Cardiovascular Exercise

Date	Length of Workout	Distance Covered	Physical Notes	Other Notes

Strength-Building and Flexibility Exercise Sessions

Date	Exercise Set Performed	Repetitions/ Weight	Physical Notes

BECOME MORE ACTIVE!

There are a good number of calories that can be burned up in a day simply by increasing the overall activity level of your life! Consider these ten suggestions:

1. Take the stairs instead of the elevator or escalator at the office, in the mall, or in the department store.

2. Park as far away from the entrance to the supermarket or store as possible. (Remember to be safe!)

3. Take a window-shopping stroll during your lunch hour.

4. Walk through a nearby park and scatter birdseed as you go. Use your morning break or lunch hour as a time to feed the neighborhood birds.

5. If you have a choice between sitting and standing . . . stand. It burns more calories.

6. Consider walking or riding a bike if your errands are near your home. If you have several errands in a close radius, park your car in a central location and walk to the various stores.

7. Rather than walk to the refrigerator during a commercial, get on a stair-stepper or mini trampoline for a quick 120-second activity break.

8. Go to the park with your children and play Frisbee.

9. Get off your bus one stop before the office and walk from there.

10. Use nonelectric appliances rather than electric ones—such as a broom, whisk, hedge clipper.

Every calorie burned in movement is a calorie that isn't stored as fat! The following chart lists some calorie-burning exercises you might consider.

ACTIVITY CALORIE COUNTER

Activity	Calories Expended Per Hour (may vary depending on environmental conditions)	
	Men (175 pounds)	Women (140 pounds)
Sitting quietly	100	80
Standing quietly	120	95
Light activities: (office work, cleaning house, and light sports such as playing golf or baseball	300	240
Moderate activities: walking briskly (3.5 mph), gardening, cycling (5.5 mph), dancing, playing basketball	460	370
Strenuous activities: jogging (9-min. mile), swimming, and playing football	730	580
Rigorous activities: running (7-min. mile), skiing, racquetball	920	740

QUESTION TO CONSIDER
Wouldn't you rather look and feel good and be healthy?

TEN IMPORTANT EXERCISE RULES

I. Never eat just before exercising.

If you eat an energy bar or drink a high-carbohydrate sports drink before you exercise, your body will use that for fuel. Chances are that during your workout you won't even get to the point where you are tapping into stored body fat.

The most effective exercise is done at least three hours *after* a person eats.

You *may,* and should, drink large amounts of water both before and during any exercise workout.

2. Do not eat right after exercising.

A person is actually burning more fat just standing around after a rigorous workout than during the first fifteen minutes of exercise! Your body will continue to rely on fat stores for fuel for up to an hour after you exercise.

Take time to cool off, shower, and get dressed and ready for the day after a workout. That time after your workout will allow your body to continue to burn up as much fat as possible before you introduce new fuel to your system. (That's when I make my famous protein drink. Well, at least my friends think it is famous.)

3. Don't compare yourself to others.

You are always going to encounter someone who is moving faster, moving with greater flexibility, or doing more repetitions with higher weights. If you compare yourself to others, you are likely to become discouraged and quit.

4. Work with an expert.

Consider the great benefits that come through working with a knowledgeable exercise physiologist or personal trainer. These professionals can help you develop an overall exercise program that is custom-tailored to your body type, physiology, and personal health goals. (Or call for my exercise videos—they teach you how to exercise in the privacy of your home.)

5. Don't confuse muscle weight with fat weight.

Many times people actually see a slight increase in their weight when they begin an exercise program. That's because muscle tissue is denser and heavier than body fat. You start gaining muscle weight at the same time you start burning body fat. Limit yourself to one trip per week to the scales. Better yet, measure body *fat loss*. That's the true measure of a "good loss." (We have body fat calipers available through my office.)

6. Get enough sleep—and sleep well.

Most people who engage in a regular exercise program discover that they sleep more soundly and more deeply. If that isn't your experience, take a look at the factors that may be keeping you from a good night's rest. Recognize that your body needs an average of eight hours of sleep every twenty-four hours. Too little sleep and you are going to feel less like exercising—in fact, you are going to feel like doing less of everything! A lack of overall energy is likely to be interpreted by you as a need for more food. The fact is you don't *need* more food, you need more sleep and more exercise. The balance between food intake, exercise output, and good sound sleep is vital!

Your body rebuilds damaged tissues and replenishes tissue fluids and nutrients while you sleep. You need to get enough rest to help this vital rejuvenation process.

7. Have the right gear.

Always wear appropriate shoes for exercising. Walking shoes for walking. Dancing shoes for dancing. And so forth. Good padding and support can help you avoid injuries and make the entire exercise experience more enjoyable.

Anticipate rain and cold weather. Have a rain parka. Dress in layers that you can put on and peel off.

If you are exercising before dawn, or after dark, be sure to wear reflective tape or clothing. White or light colors are best.

If you are a swimmer, wear goggles to protect your eyes from the chlorine. You might also want to get a pair of ear plugs.

If you are a cyclist or roller-blader, be sure to wear a helmet and protection for knees and elbows.

Make sure your exercise clothing gives you plenty of room for flexing muscles and doing a wide range of motion.

8. Exercise with others.

Make your morning exercise time a family time. If you don't have a family or if family members won't join you, find a friend who will. If you don't have a friend who will join you in exercising . . . join a gym!

9. Double task.

If you think that exercise is a waste of time, then choose to use your exercise time for mental problem-solving, watching the news, or catching up on the latest books (by listening to tapes). You can also listen to instructional or inspirational tapes while you exercise.

10. Have Fun!

Choose to have fun while you exercise. If walking or jogging around a track or your neighborhood isn't much fun for you, do something to make it fun. If you get bored doing one kind of exercise after a while, switch to another. Losing interest in exercise is often a sign of overtraining. If you've been riding a bike, try walking. If you've been walking, try swimming.

Make your exercise time interesting—make it something you look forward to doing every day!

FITTING EXERCISE INTO YOUR SCHEDULE

Are you finding it difficult to convince yourself that you have thirty to sixty minutes a day to fit exercise into your schedule? Here are a few tips:

Watch less television. (What a waste of time!)

The average American spends thirty hours a week watching TV. Carve out five of those hours for exercise!

Spend less time on the non-productive telephone chatter. (Another waste of time.)

If you insist on spending time on the phone, talk on the phone while you walk on a treadmill or ride a stationary bike.

Make a list of daily things to do that includes exercise.

Every night write down those things that you want to accomplish the next day. Put "work out" on your list!

Eat out less often.

If you eat out at restaurants more than a couple of times a week, cut back. The time you'll save waiting to be seated and served can be put to exercise use.

Get to bed earlier.

By getting to bed a half hour earlier, you should be able to get up at least a half hour earlier in the morning. There's your morning cardiovascular workout time!

Now it's your turn to be creative. Identify at least three more ways in which you can better manage your time to include daily exercise as part of your schedule:

Ways I Can Better Manage My Time to Allow for Daily Exercise

1.

2.

3.

QUESTION TO CONSIDER

What words come to mind when you hear these words: party, festivity, celebration?

ACTION STEP FOR WEEK #10

- Go to your daily planner or calendar right now and write in specific times for three cardiovascular workouts, three flexibility exercise sessions (after a cardiovascular workout or a strength-building workout), and three strength-building exercise sessions.

- Set your alarm clock for a half hour earlier tomorrow morning. When it rings, don't hit the snooze button. Rather, hit the floor, put on your shoes, and prepare to go out for a morning walk!

- Lay out all your exercise clothes (including shoes and socks) before you go to bed at night so they are ready and waiting for you when you arise.

🥞 Fat Fact

Between the ages of twenty and seventy, the average person loses approximately 30 percent of their muscle mass owing to tissue atrophy. Most of what replaces that muscle mass is *fat*.

BUILDING STRENGTH AND FLEXIBILITY

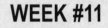

WEEK #11

CHALLENGE AND CHANGE FOR WEEK #11
Do strength-building (weight) exercises and flexibility
(stretching) exercises three to four times a week.

FAT-LOSS TIP

Eat with lean people. Most overfat people can learn a lot by eating with thin people. Watch how they push food around their plates rather than take food from plate to mouth! Watch what they order. Watch how they leave food on their plates. Adopt their ways!

STRENGTH-BUILDING EXERCISES

You need to devote at least thirty to forty-five minutes to strength-building exercises three to four times a week, regardless of your age. This type of exercise is also called *resistance* exercise. It is usually done with weights, or by doing exercises in which your own body acts as the weight. I recommend that you do this type of training every other day—which gives a day for your muscles to rebuild between workouts.

The result of muscle-building is an increase in metabolic rate, which allows you to burn up more calories just in the course of breathing and going about your daily routine. For every pound of lean muscle mass that you build into your body, you increase your metabolic rate by about fifty calories.

Lean muscle mass is absolutely necessary for efficient fat loss and the maintenance of fat loss. The achievement of lean muscle mass requires muscle growth. Even very limited amounts of strength-building exercise have been shown to increase muscle growth and overall muscle mass!

Also, since muscle tissue is responsible for 80 percent of the blood sugar uptake following a meal, every little bit of extra muscle gives a space for the body to store calories other than in fat cells!

Weight-training is actually *more* beneficial than cardiovascular exercise in burning fat. The *maximum* effect, of course, is achieved when a person does both weight-training and cardiovascular exercise on a regular schedule.

QUESTION TO CONSIDER
Are you making healthy choices regarding your work and your social life?

No Pain!

Do not ignore the signal of pain when doing strength-building exercises. If you feel a twinge of pain from a joint or ligament while doing a strength-training exercise, stop doing what triggered the pain. "No-pain, no gain" is not a good slogan for strength-training exercises. Pain in joints and ligaments is a built-in warning sign—don't ignore it.

Sets of Exercises to Do

Strength-building exercises should involve both fast-twitch and slow-twitch muscles. Each type of muscle fiber requires a different kind of exercise. Make sure you develop a personal program that covers both types of muscle groups. If you don't know the difference, ask an expert at your gym.

You will want to work with someone at a gym (or with a personal trainer) in defining a set of strength-building exercises to do. The specific exercises will vary according to the type of weights and equipment available. Virtually all good gyms have a person on staff who can help you choose exercises, give instruction in how to use the equipment safely, and recommend starting weights and numbers of repetitions.

As I also recommend flexibility exercises later in this chapter, I suggest you define a set of exercises using the following form. This will help you keep track of what you are doing from week to week, and it will also make the maintenance of your exercise log an easier task. These sets are likely to vary far less than your flexibility exercises. Occasionally, however, you may add a piece of equipment or an exercise to your set. Most of your work with weight-training will involve increasing weights and repetitions.

🥞 Fat Fact

Sixty percent of those who lose weight regain the pounds they have lost within three to five years, and a high percentage of those people actually gain back more weight. Yo-yo dieting doesn't work!

SETS OF STRENGTH-BUILDING EXERCISES

Weight Set #1

Weight Set #2

Weight Set #3

FLEXIBILITY EXERCISES

Flexibility is the ability to move muscles, joints, and bones with a full range of motion. Flexibility exercises are also called *stretching* exercises.

Flexibility exercises are vital for deterring joint and ligament problems. They also help a person maintain mobility as the person ages.

If you haven't done any flexibility training for a while, don't go overboard the first time out. Do what you can do, but don't overdo. If you can bend over and touch your knees but go no further, then work with that. Don't force yourself to go past where you can go, and *never* bounce. It takes time to increase flexibility. Be patient and stay with your program.

Be sure to stretch after doing your cardiovascular (aerobics) workout or your strength-building workout. Muscles must be thoroughly warmed up before you stretch them. Stretching after active exercise minimizes spasms, promotes relaxation of the muscles as well as the mind and nervous system, and speeds recovery by minimizing the stiffness and soreness that often go along with weight-training or aerobics exercise.

GENERAL TIPS FOR DOING
FLEXIBILITY EXERCISES

Do not stretch your muscles to the point where you feel pain. Get into a position where the target muscle (or muscle group) feels tight but is still comfortable and hold that position for ten to fifteen seconds, then release the stretch.

Second, breathe slowly and deeply while stretching—never hold your breath.

Third, of all the stretching techniques, *static* stretching is the most popular. It involves simply moving into a comfortable stretch and holding the position for the desired time. This is the safest technique.

BASIC STRETCHING EXERCISES

Here are ten beginning stretches. You'll note that each of them calls for you to hold a position from fifteen to sixty seconds. Do only what you can do comfortably. Over time, you should be able to extend the length of time you hold a position. You should be able to complete all ten of these exercises in less than twenty minutes, even doing some of them twice to stretch the muscles on both sides of your body.

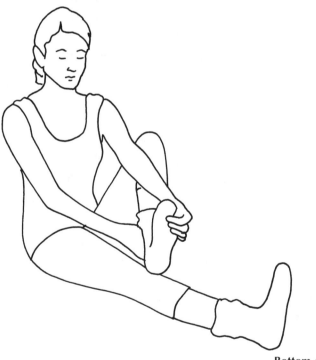

Bottom of the Foot

1. Bottom of the Foot

Sit on a mat with one leg crossed over the opposite thigh. Hold the ankle of the leg that is on top with one hand and hold the underside of your toes and ball of your foot with the other hand. Exhale and pull your toes backward toward the knee of the same leg. Hold for fifteen to sixty seconds, then relax. Do the other side.

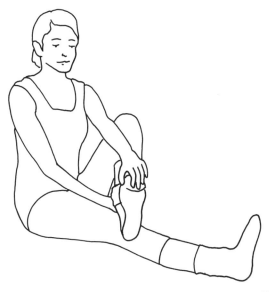

Top of the Foot

2. Top of the Foot

Sit in the same position described above. Hold the top of your toes and foot. Exhale, while slowly pulling the toes toward the ball of the foot. Hold the stretch for fifteen to sixty seconds, then relax. Do the other side.

3. Upper Back

Kneel on all fours and extend your arms forward while lowering your chest toward the floor. Exhale and extend your arms farther and press down on the floor while arching your back. (If you feel any discomfort in your upper back or shoulders, stop!) Hold the position fifteen to sixty seconds and relax.

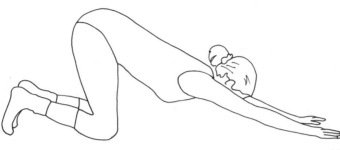

Upper back

4. Achilles Tendon

Stand upright and thrust one foot about three feet in front of the other, the toes facing directly forward, your hands on your hips, your shoulders and hips squarely forward, and your upper body upright. Bend the front leg slowly while keeping the rear knee straight. Make sure your heels are flat on the ground and your toes are facing forward. Hold for fifteen to sixty seconds, then relax. Do the other side.

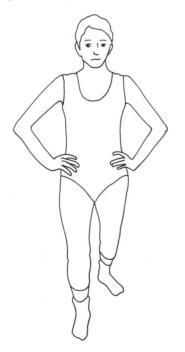

Archilles Tendon

5. Hamstrings

Sit with one leg extended straight out in front of you, your toes curled. Bring your other foot in so your heel touches your groin and your foot is flat against the opposite thigh. As you exhale, bend forward at the hip, keeping your lower back straight, your shoulders back, and your head up. Hold this position for fifteen to sixty seconds, then relax. Do the other side.

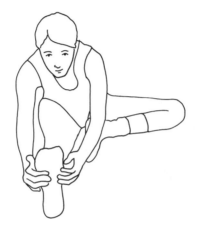

Hamstrings

6. Inner Thigh

Sit upright with your knees bent and the soles of your feet together, your heels touching or near your groin area. Hold onto your feet and rest your elbows on top of your thighs. Exhale and slowly push your legs to the floor by gently pushing down with your elbows as you pull up on your feet. Hold for fifteen to sixty seconds and relax.

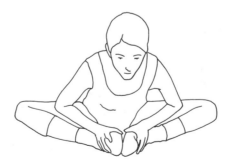

Inner Thigh

7. Hips

Stand erect and hold on to something for support with one hand while you bend one knee and bring your foot up behind you. Grab hold of that foot at the ankle with your free hand. Gently pull your foot toward your buttocks, and at the same time, keep your upper body erect, pulling up on the ankle so that the knee moves rearward. Hold for fifteen to sixty seconds, then relax. Do the other side.

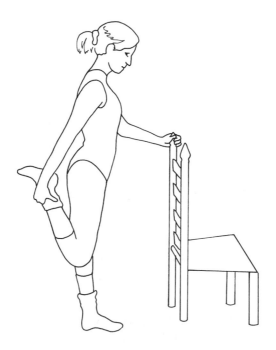

Hips

8. Buttocks and Hips

Lie flat on your back with your left leg straight and your right leg bent and raise to your chest. With your left hand grab your right knee. Your right arm should be extended perpendicular to the body. As you exhale, pull the right knee across the body so the right knee eventually touches the floor while your right arm, head, shoulders, and back remain flat. Hold for fifteen to sixty seconds, then relax. Do other side.

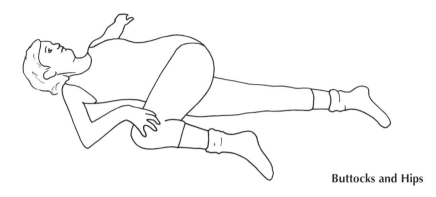

Buttocks and Hips

9. Lower Back

Kneel on your hands and knees with your toes pointed rearward. Keep your back flat and the top of head pointing directly forward. Inhale and round your back by contracting your abdominal muscles and pushing from the chest. Hold this position for fifteen to sixty seconds and relax.

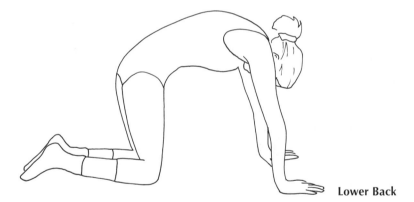

Lower Back

10. Lateral Torso

Stand upright, your feet about shoulder-width apart. Put one hand on your hip and extend the other hand overhead. As you exhale, reach overhead with your extended arm toward the opposite side of your body, keeping your shoulders and hips squarely forward. Hold this position fifteen to sixty seconds, then relax. Do other side.

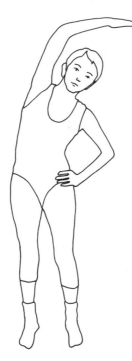

Lateral Torso

KEEPING YOUR FLEXIBILITY EXERCISE LOG

Exercise log sheets were provided in the previous chapter. I recommend that you group your flexibility exercises into sets. Define each set according to the specific exercises that you are doing.

Based upon the flexibility exercises described previously, the following examples of sets of exercises might be labeled "Set #1" and "Set #2" for your first week of flexibility workouts.

Set #1

Bottom of the Foot
Top of the Foot
Upper Back
Achilles Tendon
Hamstrings

Set #2:

Inner Thigh

Hips

Buttocks and Hips

Lower Back

Lateral Torso

The following space is provided for you to identify up to twelve exercise sets as you progress during the coming weeks—doing different combinations of stretching exercises with more repetitions at each workout.

EXERCISE SETS DEFINED

Exercise Set #1

Exercise Set #2

Exercise Set #3

Exercise Set #4

Exercise Set #5

Exercise Set #6

Exercise Set #7

Exercise Set #8

Exercise Set #9

Exercise Set #10

Exercise Set #11

Exercise Set #12

Feel free to define additional flexibility exercise sets as you branch out to more difficult ones or combine these exercises in new ways.

🥞 Fat Fact

After glucose has been converted to fat, it can *not* be converted back to glucose. One of the only ways to get rid of fat is to burn it off through consistent cardiovascular and strength-building exercise!

15 SPECIFIC EXERCISES FOR
A FLATTER TUMMY

The tummy area is one of the areas of the body that many obese people find problematic as they lose weight.

Fat tends to leave the abdomen before it leaves other areas, which can leave a significant amount of flab that needs tightening. Some of this happens over time as the body adjusts to collapsed fat cells in the abdominal cavity. Exercises, however, can greatly speed up this adjustment.

Keep in mind that these tummy-tightening exercises do not work overnight. Maintaining a flat stomach also requires *time*. The exercises, however, are relatively easy and if you stay with them, you will definitely be helped.

Along with a sleeker look, you should also feel increased abdominal strength within a few weeks, perhaps even a few days. Be encouraged, but don't expect others to comment on your new physique. You probably won't *see* a flatness to your stomach for a month or more. When your waistline starts to shrink—as it inevitably will if you stick with the exercises and eating programs—you will first be able to tell your stomach is flatter because of the way your clothes fit.

Also recognize that the older you are and the less you've been exercising in the past, the longer it will take for your exercising to show on your body. However, you will likely *feel* the benefits of the strength-building and flexibility exercises almost immediately.

Following are fifteen exercises. Look closely at the diagrams and slowly try out these exercises to be certain you are doing them correctly. Once through the entire set of fifteen is sufficient on your first day of exercising these muscles.

On the second day, do the first eight exercises—two times each. On the third day, do the second seven exercises—two times each.

Continue this alternating pattern for the first week. Then increase to three repetitions of the first seven and three repetitions of the second eight, alternating days for another week or two.

During the next several weeks, try four repetitions of the first five exercises, four reps of the second five, and four reps of the third five exercises. Add a repetition every couple of weeks until you are doing about eight reps of each of three sets of exercises. Your ultimate goal is a dozen reps of three exercises a day, which means that in a five-day exercise week, you are only doing each exercise one time, but for twelve reps.

Don't get too hung up on when exactly you should add more reps and decrease the number of exercises you are doing. Let your body be the guide for that. Just know that your ultimate goal is twelve reps a day of three exercises.

1. From Ceiling to Floor

Stand with your back twelve to twenty-four inches from a wall, feet shoulder-width apart, arms stretched overhead, elbows straight, hands shoulder-width apart. Bend back and touch the wall with your fingernails, keeping your knees and elbows as straight as possible. Return to the starting position and immediately bend forward and touch the floor, your knees still as straight as possible Return to the starting position. This is one repetition.

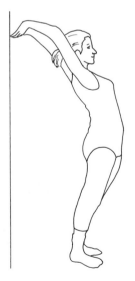

From Ceiling to Floor

2. Chest Pull

Lie on your back, your arms stretched overhead against the floor and your buttocks resting on the floor. Pull both knees up as close as possible to your chest. Then extend one leg straight out, parallel to the floor, but not quite touching it. The other leg should remain bent, drawn as close to the chest as possible. Then draw the extended leg back close to the chest, and extend the second leg straight out. Draw the second knee back, while again extending the first leg. Continue this bicycle-peddling type motion until you have moved each leg out and back four times. That is one repetition.

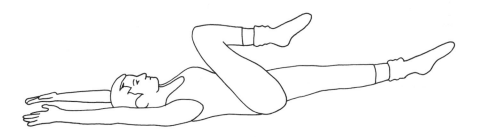

Chest Pull

3. Abdominal Crunch

Lie on your back, legs bent, with your knees pointed toward the ceiling, feet flat on the floor, hands on your chest, fingers interlocked. Exhale as you rise up from the waist up, moving only about three to six inches above the floor. Inhale as you lower back to the starting position. This is one repetition. (You may find it helpful to place your feet under a heavy piece of furniture, such as a dresser or couch, to help you keep your feet in place.)

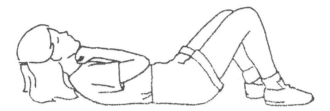

Abdominal Crunch

4. Body Twist

Stand with your feet comfortably more than shoulder-width apart, your arms stretched sideward and parallel to the floor, your elbows straight. Keep your feet planted firmly, and slowly twist the trunk of your body as far to the right as possible. Stretch, pulling the right arm back and pulling the left arm around to the right as far as it will comfortably go. Snap back to the starting position and place your hands on your hips. Return to your starting position and repeat the move to the left. This is one repetition.

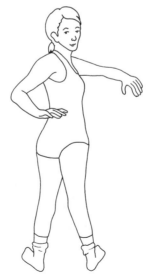

Body Twist

5. Swing Beyond the Legs

Stand with your feet comfortably more than shoulder-width apart, your arms overhead, your elbows straight, and your hands shoulder-width apart. Rapidly swing your upper body forward and down, while bending your knees slightly. Reach back through the legs, and touch the ground as far back as possible. Swing your upper body back up and stop suddenly, almost jerking to a stop at the starting point. This is one repetition.

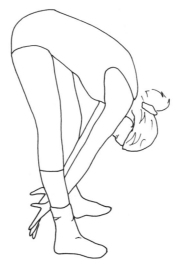

Swing Beyond

6. Upside-Down V

Lie on your stomach with your hands above your hips and close to your sides, your elbows pointed at the ceiling, your palms on the floor with your fingers pointed toward your shoulders. Keep your feet on the ground and raise your head, shoulders, and chest as high as possible, arching your back. Then raise your rear high (keeping your hands and feet in place), until your body forms an inverted V shape. Bearing your weight on your hands and feet, and keeping your knees and elbows straight, remain in this V shape and pull in your stomach until it feels tight. Hold this position for up to six seconds. Lower your rear to the original arched position, then back to the starting position. This is one repetition.

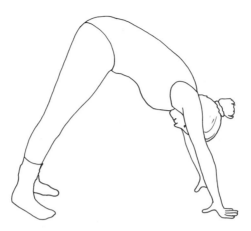

Upside Down V

7. Upper Body Twist

Sit with your legs bent, knees pointed toward the ceiling, feet flat on the floor (perhaps with your feet under a heavy piece of furniture as in Exercise 3.) Put your hands on the back of your head, your fingers interlocked. Then lean back until your upper body is at a forty-five-degree angle. Twist your upper body as far as possible to the left, then to the right, and then return forward. Finally, lean back to your original upright torso position. This is one repetition. Twist to the left the first half of your repetitions, then to the right the second half of your repetitions. In other words, if you are doing ten reps, twist to the left for the first five, then to the right for the second five.

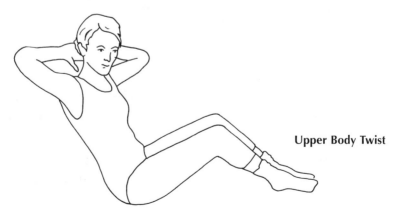

Upper Body Twist

8. Lean Over

Stand with your feet shoulder-width apart, your hands on your hips. Reach over your head with your left hand, touching your right ear. Bend sideward to the right, sliding your right hand as far as possible down the right leg and stretching your left side as much as possible without pain. Do not allow yourself to reach forward or backward in order to stretch farther down with your right hand. Return to the starting position and repeat to the left. This is one repetition.

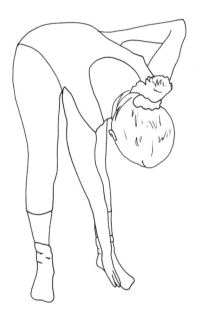

Lean Over

9. Legs Over Head

Lie on your back, your legs straight and together, your arms stretched overhead against the floor. Try to keep your legs straight as you lift them up together and bring them over your head, continuing back and downward until your toes are as close to the floor above your head as possible. Return your legs to the starting position, reversing the motion you have just done, keeping your legs straight and together. This is one repetition. Be careful. This is a difficult movement!

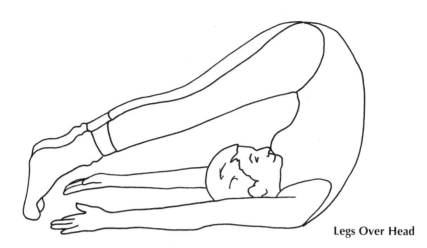

Legs Over Head

10. Cross-Over Abdominal Crunch

This is the same basic exercise as Exercise 3, except that as you raise up, twist your trunk slightly toward one side of your body. Return to the starting position. This is one repetition. Twist to the other side on the second half of your reps.

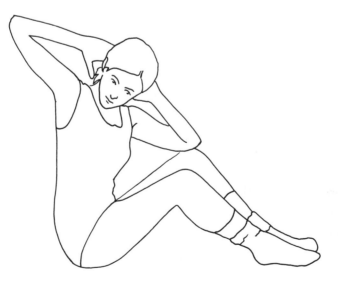

Cross-Over Abdominal Crunch

11. Tree in the Wind

Stand with your feet comfortably more than shoulder-width apart, your arms straight overhead, your elbows straight, your palms toward the ceiling, with your fingers interlocked. Bend sideward to the right as far as possible, stretching your left side. Straighten and bend immediately back, stretching your arms and shoulders backward. Straighten and bend forward, touching or nearly touching your palms to the floor. Keep your knees straight throughout the exercise. Return to your starting position. This is one repetition. Change directions, bending to the right for the first half of your repetitions, to the left during the second half of your repetitions.

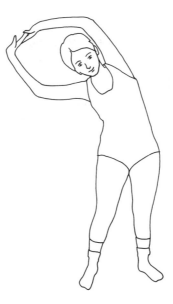

Tree in the Wind

12. Make a Lazy U

Lie on your stomach, your hands clasped in the small of your back, your legs straight. Raise your head, chest, and shoulders as high as possible. At the same time, raise your feet and legs together to their maximum height. Hold momentarily, then lower to the starting position. This is one repetition.

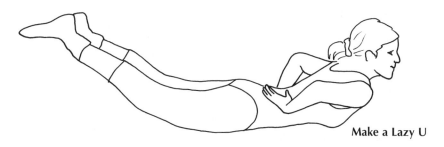

Make a Lazy U

13. Hip Lift

Stand with your feet shoulder-width apart, your arms at your sides, your elbows straight. Lift your right hip sideward toward your right shoulder, allowing your right foot to come off the ground slightly. *Do not* move the right leg sideward. Also do not intentionally lift your right foot; just *allow* it to come up as you intentionally lift your right hip. Return to the starting position. Repeat for the same side as one repetition. The movement should be done twice in success on the left side as one repetition. Do the first half of your reps on one side, the second half on the other side. Again, if you're doing ten reps, do five reps (ten hip lifts) on one side and then five reps (ten hip lifts) on the left side.

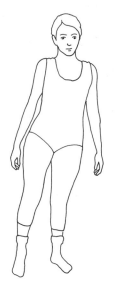

Hip Lift

171

14. Cross-Over Toe Touch

Stand with your feet comfortably more than shoulder-width apart, your hands on your hips. Reach sideward, then straight overhead with your right arm. Stretch your right side thoroughly, continuing the movement of your right arm and your upper body to the left and then downward. Remain stretched at the shoulder as long as you can maintain the sideward motion and keep the sideward motion as long as possible. Allow yourself to twist forward at the waist at the end of the movement and, keeping the legs straight, attempt to touch the floor outside the left foot. Return through the same path to the starting position. Repeat the movement, with your left arm toward the right. This is one repetition.

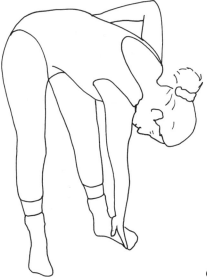

Cross-Over Toe Touch

15. Legs to the Sky

Lie on your back, your feet together, your toes pointed, your arms stretched overhead against the floor, your elbows straight, your hands shoulder-width apart. Raise your legs, keeping them straight until they are vertical. Lower your legs slowly to the starting position. This is one repetition.

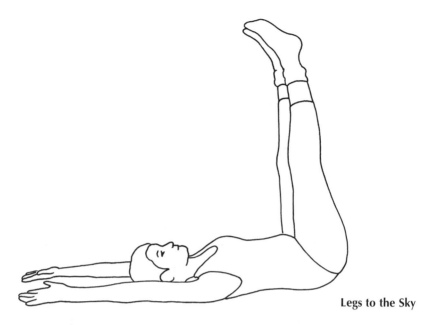

Legs to the Sky

You should not sweat profusely in doing these exercises. If you feel stiff or sore after the first day—or any day, for that matter—try these methods of relief:

1. Stand in a warm shower or soak in a tub of warm water. *Gently* massage the stiff or sore area.

2. Reduce either the number of exercises in your workout or the number of repetitions per exercise, or both.

3. If a specific exercise seems too difficult or causes pain, soreness, or stiffness, leave it out. After several months of doing the aerobic, weight-training, and flexibility exercises that are part of your more generalized fat-loss plan, see if you can do them. If yes, fine. If not, do those you can do and don't worry about the rest.

EXERCISING AWAY A DOUBLE CHIN

A second area of the anatomy that many obese people find problematic is the chin. Suddenly, it seems, they discover they have a double chin.

Just as with exercising the stomach area, the good news about a double chin is that specific exercises can help tighten the muscle tissues involved. The exercises don't work overnight and you need to remain diligent in doing them, but they do work. In fact, those who have done these exercises claim that a double chin can be virtually eliminated in a matter of weeks.

These chin exercises, which are recommended by William Hintermister in his book *How to Get Rid of Your Double Chin in Just Six Weeks* (1982), should be performed slowly, smoothly, and without strain.

If you feel any signs of discomfort at overdoing an exercise, stop exercising and head for the shower. Stand under a stream of warm water for about ten minutes, slowly turning your head from side to side to get the full benefit of the warm water.

As you do each of these exercises, breathe rhythmically through your nose, using your diaphragm. Inhale for three counts, hold two counts, exhale four counts. For each exercise sit in a comfortable chair or stool in front of a mirror.

Chin and Neck Swivel

Sit up straight with your shoulders relaxed. Lift your chin, pointing it toward the ceiling. Pull your head back. Slowly turn your head five times in each direction.

Then rotate your head slowly clockwise. Sweep your chin across the top of your chest to your shoulder area. Continue by lifting up your chin and head to complete one rotation. Do five rotations in a clockwise direction and then repeat five times in a counterclockwise direction.

Pause to take a couple of breaths and then repeat the entire exercise.

Bishop's Bite

Pivot your head upward until your neck is taught. Jut out your chin. Without moving your head, drop your chin down as far as possible and open your mouth as wide as you can. Keep your head still with your jaw jutted out. Lift your jaw and touch your teeth together gently. Then lower and raise your jaw rapidly. Don't hit your teeth together hard. Do this ten times. Relax for two breaths and repeat ten times.

Chin Isometric

Pivot your chin upward several inches, clenching your teeth firmly together in a natural bite position.

Place the back of your right hand firmly against your throat, just above the adam's apple. Push with the tip of your tongue against the bottom of your mouth behind your lower front teeth. Keep your hand firmly in place to provide resistance. Increase the downward tongue pressure gradually and hold for six seconds. Hold at almost full pressure for six more seconds. Slowly relax your tongue pressure and rest. Take two full breaks and repeat twice, breathing in between.

Vacuum Pull

Breathe twice. Keep your teeth in the natural bite position while lifting your chin up and out until your neck is taught. With your lips tightly closed, attempt to suck air into your mouth. Maintain an inward sucking pressure to the count of ten. Relax for three breaths. Repeat.

Jaw Lift

Lift your chin up and slightly out until your neck is taut. Open your mouth and lower your jaw as far as possible. Jut out your jaw and raise it very slowly in a "steam shovel digging" fashion. Hold your head still and concentrate on lifting with only the muscles of your chin and neck.

Lift your lower teeth over your upper teeth and your lower lip over your upper lip. Attempt to touch your nose with your bottom lip. Hold for one breath. Relax. Repeat this entire exercise ten times.

After doing this exercise regularly for two weeks, you can improve your results by placing your hands on your breastbone, pulling and holding your skin tightly as you perform the movements.

Shoulder Touches

Position your lower lip over your upper lip. Position your lower teeth over your upper teeth. Concentrate on your chin muscles. Try to touch your chin to your left shoulder. Then try to touch your left ear to your left shoulder. Do this five times to the left, then five times to the right. Don't grind your teeth. Relax and take two breaths. Then repeat.

Tongue and Chin

Jut your chin out and up until your neck is all the way back resting against your shoulders. With your teeth together in a natural bite position, lift your lower lip over your upper lip by moving your chin muscles. With the tip of your tongue, press against the bottom of your mouth behind the lower front teeth. Breathe correctly through your nose. Increase the pressure with your tongue gradually to the count of eight until you are pushing with maximum force. Relax for two breaths. Repeat.

ACTION STEPS FOR WEEK #11

- Do a flexibility exercise work-out after your next cardiovascular work-out.

- Purchase a small set of hand weights (two pounds is a good starting weight) that you can carry with you while you are doing your aerobics exercise.

- Treat yourself to a massage or a half hour in a whirlpool bath or hot tub after your first strength-building work-out.

- I really suggest you order my workout videos from my office: 1-800-726-1834. Videos are available for men or women—beginning, intermediate, and advanced levels.

QUESTION TO CONSIDER
Do your food attitudes parallel your attitudes toward love, money, and sex?

GIVING YOUR BODY *ALL* THE NUTRIENTS IT NEEDS

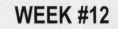

WEEK #12

CHALLENGE AND CHANGE FOR WEEK #12
Take supplements daily to help fight fat
and give your body all the nutrients it needs.

Fat-Loss Tip

Make certain that you immediately rehydrate your muscle cells by drinking sufficient water after exercise.

ALL THE NUTRIENTS IN
SUFFICIENT QUANTITY

The human body needs forty-five essential nutrients for good health. These are nutrients that must be taken into the body from an outside source. Of these forty-five nutrients, twenty are minerals, fifteen are vitamins, eight are essential amino acids (building blocks for proteins), and two are essential fatty acids. We need sufficient quantities of these nutrients every day for optimal health and maximum fat loss.

Food alone cannot supply all the basic vitamins and minerals needed by the average person on a fat-loss program. Exercise creates a different level of need for certain nutrients—the same for a fat-loss eating plan. A person needs far more than the Recommended Dietary Allowances (RDA) of vitamins and minerals—which means that a one-a-day pill can never be sufficient.

Virtually all people on a fat-loss program need to take supplements of vitamins and minerals on a daily basis.

FIVE GENERAL RULES FOR
TAKING SUPPLEMENTS

1. Other than vitamin C, do not take megadoses of any supplement for a prolonged period of time without consulting a physician. You want an adequate amount of nutrients, but not prolonged megadoses!

2. Do not depend solely on fat-burning supplements. Fat-burning

supplements only work if your exercise and nutrition program is in line.

3. Avoid any tendency to skip a workout or blow your eating plan and then take a megadose of supplements. Supplements are never a replacement for a good, clean diet, intense workouts, and sufficient water to keep the body flushed of any toxins that may be generated as a by-product of fat-burning processes.

4. Always buy supplements from a reputable dealer. Make sure the products are clearly labeled as to their ingredients and recommended dosages.

5. If you have any doubt about taking a supplement, call my office.

SUPPLEMENTS THAT HELP WITH FAT LOSS

These are my top ten picks of fat-loss nutrients that can be taken in supplemental form.

1. Chromium Picolinate

Chromium has been shown to reduce sugar cravings by improving the metabolism of simple carbohydrates. It is an extremely valuable supplement for those with diabetes or hypoglycemia because it helps to regulate blood sugar levels. Normal dosage is two hundred to six hundred mcg daily. Look for chromium picolinate or chromium polynicotinate.

2. Lecithin

This can be purchased in granule or capsule form. Lecithin is a fat emulsifier—it breaks down fat so it can be readily removed from the body. If you are using granules, take 1 tablespoon three times a day before meals. In capsule form, the dosage is one thousand two hundred milligrams three times a day before meals. The best source of lecithin is soybean oil. It's a great source of two of the hardest-to-find B vitamins: choline and inositol. Not only that, it's loaded in vitamin E. I suggest adding lecithin to your morning protein shake.

3. L-Arginine

4. L-Ornithine

5. L-Lysine

These three nutrients plus a fifty milligram tablet of vitamin B6 and a one hundred milligram tablet of vitamin C makes an excellent "bedtime cocktail" of nutrients that are especially beneficial in helping your body burn fat all night long

Take five hundred milligrams of each, or as directed on the label before bedtime, on an empty stomach with water or juice. Do not use milk with these amino acids.

These amino acids should not be used by those who have diabetes, ocular or brain herpes infections, pituitary dysfunction, or cancer.

6. L-Carnitine

This amino acid, which is found in many foods and especially meat, helps ensure optimal metabolism of fat. It has the ability to break up fat deposits and it aids in weight loss. It is an important supplement to consider if your fat loss is exceeding one and a half pounds a week. If you take it in supplement form, be sure to take it with meals. Recommended dosage is five hundred milligrams daily.

Make certain that you take L-Carnitine. The use of D-Carnitine or D-L-Carnitine has been associated with some severe side effects. Check the label!

7. L-Glutamine (not glutamic acid, which is toxic)

This nutrient lessens carbohydrate cravings. Use as directed on the label.

L-Glutamine nourishes the cells of the immune system. It is an essential nitrogen transporter that allows ammonia to be removed from the body, and it is one of the main building blocks for one of the most powerful antioxidants produced in the body: gluthathione (made from glutamine, cysteine, and glycine). Of all the amino acids, glutamine appears to be by far the most important one in helping muscle cells to stay hydrated and continue to grow (as opposed to becoming dehydrated, shriveled, and wasted away).

The best time to take glutamine is right after exercise.

8. Zinc

Zinc enhances the effectiveness of insulin and boosts the immune system. Use zinc gluconate for best absorption. Recommended dosage is sixty milligrams a day. Check the label on your general mineral supplement. If it has eighty milligrams of zinc, do not add additional zinc. Zinc, however, is water-soluble and therefore, if too much is taken, it is readily excreted in the urine.

Zinc should be taken on an empty stomach at night before bedtime.

Zinc must be taken in proportionate levels to copper, iron, and chromium. You likely will be able to find a supplement that balances zinc with copper, iron, and chromium. I use a powdered multivitamin in my shake. Its much easier for the body to absorb than a pill.

9. Magnesium

Magnesium is related to more than three hundred different chemical reactions in the body. It promotes muscle strength, endurance, and relaxation, and it is vitally important for protein synthesis.

Magnesium deficiency has been linked to heart disease.

Make sure your eating plan includes foods rich in magnesium, such as whole grains, beans, sesame seeds, and a limited quantity of nuts (such as blanched almonds and cashews). Halibut and sole are fish high in magnesium. Avocados are also a great source for this mineral.

Magnesium supplements are also available. You should go easy on supplements at first because, in excessive amounts, they can cause diarrhea. Stay away from cheaper, inorganic forms such as magnesium chloride or carbonate. Instead, take the supplements that have the words *malate, fumarate, citrate, taurate,* or *glycinate* associated with magnesium—these forms are better absorbed, tolerated, and utilized in the body.

I recommend four hundred to five hundred milligrams of magnesium. It should be taken on an empty stomach at night before bedtime.

Magnesium is a mineral that works in balance with calcium. Too much calcium can block magnesium absorption. Vitamin B6 works with magnesium in many of the energy-producing reactions.

10. Hydroxycitric Acid (HCA)

This substance is extracted from the rind of the fruit of the *Garcinia cambogia* tree. Not only does HCA suppress hunger but it helps to prevent the body from turning carbohydrate calories into fat. Follow directions on the label.

Also Good . . .

- Conjugated Linoleic Acid (CLA) (I take these daily.)

- Xylitol

- Synephrine

- L-Tyrosine (Do not take this, however, if you use MAO inhibitors, have cardiac arrhythmias, psychosis, preexisting malignant melanoma-type cancer, or have a violent temper.)

- HMB (B-hydroxy b-methyl butyrate monohydrate)

- Creatine Monohydrate

- Calcium (Calcium needs to be taken in balance with magnesium.)

- Boron (Raisins and onions are good food sources of boron.)

For more details on these supplements, see the *Maximum Fat Loss* book.

🥞 Fat Fact

One out of every three Americans is at least 20 percent overweight and about three out of four Americans are heavier than their optimal weight.

HERBS THAT HELP WITH FAT LOSS

In addition to the nutrients described above, these herbs can help with fat loss:

Herbal Diuretic Teas

Alfalfa, corn silk, dandelion, gravel root, horsetail, hydrangea, hyssop, juniper berries, oat straw, parsley, seawrack, thyme, uva ursi, white ash, and yarrow can be used in tea form as a natural diuretic.

Aloe Vera

This juice improves digestion and cleanses the digestive tract.

Herbs That Aid Digestion

Butcher's broom, cardamom, cayenne, cinnamon, *Garcinia cambogia*, ginger, green tea, and mustard seed are thermogenic herbs. Do not use cinnamon in large quantities if you are pregnant or think you might become pregnant.

Herbs That Improve Thyroid Function

Bladderwrack, borage seed, hawthorn berry, and sarsaparilla stimulate the adrenal glands and improve thyroid function.

Fennel

Fennel removes mucus and fat from the intestinal tract and is a natural appetite suppressant.

Fenugreek

This herb helps dissolve fat in the liver.

Siberian Ginseng

This herb aids in moving fluids and nutrients throughout the body and reduces the stress often associated with acquiring new eating habits.

Do not use this herb if you have hypoglycemia, high blood pressure, or a heart disorder.

Yohimbe Bark Extract

In women, this extract appears to decrease fat synthesis and increase the release of fatty acids from fat stores.

St. John's Wort

This plant seems to decrease food cravings and help a person avoid food binges.

Chlorella

A small, one-celled algae, chlorellais a powerhouse of vitamins, minerals, and protein. It is an excellent product to take to help detoxify your body. It should be taken with at least eight ounces of water.

Wheat Grass

Wheat grass is high in fiber and protein. It contains chlorophyll and other nutrients that are often associated with deep green and leafy vegetables. When taken before meals with a large glass of water, wheat grass expands at least fifteen times its original volume to help a person feel full.

Barley

Young barley can be juiced to yield a product that is a rich source of vitamins, minerals, and enzymes. It is especially rich in vitamins B1 and B12 and is high in vitamin C, carotene, and calcium. It is available in tablets or granules.

Kelp

Kelp acts on obesity by helping to normalize thyroid gland function.

QUESTION TO CONSIDER
In what ways have you used your obesity as an excuse for not doing certain things?

GENERAL SUPPLEMENTS THAT
ARE VERY HELPFUL

A mounting pile of scientific research is showing that vitamins, especially vitamin E and vitamin C, beta carotene, and minerals such as zinc and selenium, may offer significant protection against cancer, atherosclerosis, birth defects, cataracts, and other conditions.

I recommend a person take sufficient quantities of these vitamins daily. I can only touch the surface concerning supplements in this book. Please order my tape series *Forever Fit* for extensive literature and information on this topic.

Vitamin C with Bioflavonoids

Vitamin C actually helps to speed up a slow metabolism and assists in normalizing glandular function. General recommended dosage for those on a fat-loss program is three thousand to six thousand milligrams daily. Space out your vitamin C. I recommend taking a thousand milligrams with each of six meals each day. When I have been under a lot of stress, I take an extra dose of vitamin C at bedtime.

Vitamin B complex

The B vitamins help greatly to promote good digestion. Recommended dosage is fifty milligrams three times a day. Riboflavin (B2) helps the body to be more efficient in burning calories. You may want to take an extra fifty milligrams three times a day beyond what is in the fifty milligrams B complex. Niacin (B3) lessens sugar cravings and it can also be taken as fifty milligrams three times a day—but do not exceed this amount and do not take niacin if you have a liver disorder, gout, or high blood pressure. Vitamin B6 boosts the metabolism and an additional five hundred and nine milligrams three times a day is helpful. The same for vitamin B12—fifty milligrams three times a day—to help in proper digestion and absorption.

Choline and Inositol are part of the B-vitamin family. Both of these help the body burn fat and they can often be purchased as separate supplements. Use as directed on the label of the product you purchase.

Take your B vitamins in the morning with your protein shake.

Gelatin

Choose Grays Lake kosher unflavored gelatin, not the sugar-laden Jell-O, nor the sugar-free Jell-O that is enhanced with sweeteners. Gelatin is made from animal collagen, which is an essential structural protein that forms an important part of bones, tendons, and connective tissues. It contains an exceptionally high content of two amino acids that play an important role in collagen formation in the body: proline and glycine. Mix two tablespoons daily in your morning protein drink. (If you are unable to find this product, we carry this product through our office.)

Flaxseed Oil

This oil helps reduce pain associated with any type of inflammatory condition, including joint problems. If you have these problems, consider taking flaxseed oil as part of your daily dose of essential fatty acids. Be aware, however, that too much flax seed oil can interfere with your fat-burning metabolism.

Vitamin E and Selenium

Excellent for your heart! I take at least eight hundred IUs every night.

Pygnogenol

An excellent antioxidant that helps build your immune system.

CoEnzyme Q10

Excellent for the heart. I take 100mg daily.

🥞 Fat Fact

Obesity has been linked to arthritis, gout, and even cataracts.

SOME PRODUCTS YOU SHOULD NOT TAKE

There are some things you should *never* take into your body:

Alcohol

Not in any form. Not in any amount.

Cigarette Smoke or Smokeless Tobacco Products

Nicotine causes far more harm than good. The same for the tar in cigarettes and smokeless tobacco.

Steroids

Do *not* take steroids to try to build up muscle mass in your body. Steroids do help muscles grow faster, but the results of too much steroid use can be devastating. Most steroid compounds are illegal—the buying, selling, and using of anabolic steroids are all crimes. Problems in the human body seem to range from severe acne to water retention, from the development of gynecomastia (build-up of breast tissue in the mammary glands of men) to premature hair loss. More serious health problems have also been implicated, including premature death. The risks just aren't worth any short-term results you might experience.

Ephedrine

This stuff is dangerous. Some reports have linked ephedrine to both strokes and high blood pressure in susceptible people or those who overdose. Those with preexisting conditions including prostate enlargement, cardiovascular disease, thyroid diseases, and diabetes should not touch it.

Ephedrine is banned in several states but its herbal parent, ephedra—or as it's known in the Orient, *ma huang*—is still widely available. Ephedra is an herb that should not never be used if you experience heart palpitations, elevations in blood pressure, or headaches.

L-Phenylalanine

Even small doses of this can cause permanent brain damage. As explained in the *Maximum Fat Loss* book, L-Phenylalanine is one of the primary components of aspartame, the artificial sweetener.

L-Phenylalanine is especially dangerous if you are taking an MAO inhibitor (antidepressants often have these), as well as to those who have cardiac arrhythmias, hypertension, the genetic disease PKU, psychosis, existing pigmented malignant melanoma-type cancer, or a violent temper.

Testosterone

Testosterone can boost muscle mass and sexual drive. But it can also cause liver damage and accelerate the growth and proliferation of prostate cancer cells. It has been linked to prostate tumors, a blocking of sperm production, and a reduction in HDL (good) cholesterol. We do not know the long-term effects of taking testosterone supplements. Put your money into things that *work,* not things that *could* cause side effects.

Also, use caution in taking thermogenic stack supplements. Read the label for precautions. Remember always that your body will develop a resistance to any thermogenic product—if you use one of these supplements, you must vary the dosage and the days it is taken.

QUESTION TO CONSIDER

After reading *Maximum Fat Loss,* what new insights do you have into *why* diets have not worked for you in the past?

YOUR NUTRIENTS SHOPPING LIST

Make a list of the supplements that you know you need to take. As a starter, I have listed those things that I take daily or which are part of the protein drinks I make each morning.

- vitamin C

- vitamin B complex (with sufficient amounts of all the B vitamins)

- vitamin E and Selenium

- zinc

- pycnogenol

- coenzyme Q10

- chromium (and vanadyl sulfate in a complex)

- calcium-Magnesium

- gelatin (Grays Lake)

- pure cod liver oil

_____

_____

_____

_____

_____

_____

_____

_____

_____

ACTION STEPS FOR WEEK #12

- Do not eat foods that are steeped in preservatives.

- Do not eat pork.

- Do not eat shellfish.

- Remember, no bread of any type.

🥞 Fat Fact

As Americans, we've gained a whopping twelve pounds per person, on the average, in just the last decade.

TYING IT
ALL TOGETHER

What might a daily routine look like for the person who is pursuing maximum fat loss?

Here's a sample day:

A MAXIMUM FAT LOSS DAY

6:00 A.M.   Arise and drink 16 ounces of pure water.

6:30 A.M.   Do fifteen to twenty-five minutes of aerobic exercise.

7:00 A.M.   Do twenty minutes of strength-building exercise. Drink sixteen ounces of water.

7:20 A.M.   Do an additional ten to fifteen minutes of cardiovascular exercise. Drink eight ounces of pure water.

8:00–9:00 A.M.
Let your body burn fat during this cool-down period.

9:00 a.m.   Take one tablespoon of cod liver oil, three Conjugated Linoleic Acid (CLA) pills with eight ounces of water.

9:05 A.M.   Make and drink a protein-powder drink mixed with fruit (such as banana or strawberry). You may want to mix two servings and drink only half.

10:30 A.M. Drink sixteen ounces of water and then eat a protein energy bar (two hundred calories) and an apple or other piece of low-glycemic fruit. Eat *no* high-glycemic carbs and *no* bread. Instead, you might drink half of a double-portion protein drink you made earlier in the day and refrigerated. (If you are going to divide your shake, be sure to add only half of the gelatin to the first batch, and then add the second half of the gelatin to the second batch just before reblending and drinking.)

12:30 P.M. Lunch on a six ounce chicken breast and steamed low-glycemic-index vegetables and sixteen ounces of water.

3:00 P.M. Snack on some fat-free yogurt and half a pear with sixteen ounces of water.

5:30 P.M. Dine on six ounces of chicken, turkey, or fish, with a salad (fat-free dressing) and/or low-glycemic-index steamed vegetables. Drink sixteen ounces of water.

8:00 P.M. Snack on half a cup of nonfat cottage cheese or non-fat yogurt.

10:00 P.M. Take evening supplements at bedtime but eat *no* food. At night, I take at least eight hundred IU of vitamin E and selenium (together), eighty milligrams of zinc, pygnogenol, one hundred milligrams of Co-Enzyme Q10, one thousand milligrams of vitamin C and Atrie Aloe.

Take B vitamins in the morning with your protein shake—the shake is loaded with nutrients so it should provide most of what you need. If you need recipes for healthy and delicious meals, order my wife's cookbook from my office.

YOUR DAILY SCHEDULE

Below is a blank daily schedule for you to complete. Rather than identify specific food items for meals, you may want to simply put the meal number (1 to 6) and perhaps put an emphasis on protein for the first and last meals of the day.

Take one thousand milligrams with each meal and at bedtime.

Only one week's worth of forms are in this workbook. You should feel free to duplicate this schedule as many times as you desire. I recommend that you put it into your log binder under a tab labeled SCHEDULE.

IDEAL DAILY SCHEDULE

Time	Activity (meal, exercise, or supplements)
A.M.	
5:30	
6:00	
6:30	
7:00	
7:30	
8:00	
8:30	
9:00	
9:30	
10:00	
10:30	
11:00	
11:30	
P.M.	
12:00	
12:30	
1:00	
1:30	
2:00	
2:30	
3:00	
3:30	
4:00	
4:30	
5:00	
5:30	
6:00	
6:30	
7:00	
7:30	
8:00	
8:30	
9:00	
9:30	
10:00	
10:30	
11:00	

IDEAL DAILY SCHEDULE

Time	Activity (meal, exercise, or supplements)
A.M.	
5:30	
6:00	
6:30	
7:00	
7:30	
8:00	
8:30	
9:00	
9:30	
10:00	
10:30	
11:00	
11:30	
P.M.	
12:00	
12:30	
1:00	
1:30	
2:00	
2:30	
3:00	
3:30	
4:00	
4:30	
5:00	
5:30	
6:00	
6:30	
7:00	
7:30	
8:00	
8:30	
9:00	
9:30	
10:00	
10:30	
11:00	

IDEAL DAILY SCHEDULE

Time	Activity (meal, exercise, or supplements)
A.M.	
5:30	
6:00	
6:30	
7:00	
7:30	
8:00	
8:30	
9:00	
9:30	
10:00	
10:30	
11:00	
11:30	
P.M.	
12:00	
12:30	
1:00	
1:30	
2:00	
2:30	
3:00	
3:30	
4:00	
4:30	
5:00	
5:30	
6:00	
6:30	
7:00	
7:30	
8:00	
8:30	
9:00	
9:30	
10:00	
10:30	
11:00	

IDEAL DAILY SCHEDULE

Time	Activity (meal, exercise, or supplements)
A.M.	
5:30	
6:00	
6:30	
7:00	
7:30	
8:00	
8:30	
9:00	
9:30	
10:00	
10:30	
11:00	
11:30	
P.M.	
12:00	
12:30	
1:00	
1:30	
2:00	
2:30	
3:00	
3:30	
4:00	
4:30	
5:00	
5:30	
6:00	
6:30	
7:00	
7:30	
8:00	
8:30	
9:00	
9:30	
10:00	
10:30	
11:00	

IDEAL DAILY SCHEDULE

Time	Activity (meal, exercise, or supplements)
A.M.	
5:30	
6:00	
6:30	
7:00	
7:30	
8:00	
8:30	
9:00	
9:30	
10:00	
10:30	
11:00	
11:30	
P.M.	
12:00	
12:30	
1:00	
1:30	
2:00	
2:30	
3:00	
3:30	
4:00	
4:30	
5:00	
5:30	
6:00	
6:30	
7:00	
7:30	
8:00	
8:30	
9:00	
9:30	
10:00	
10:30	
11:00	

IDEAL DAILY SCHEDULE

Time	Activity (meal, exercise, or supplements)
A.M.	
5:30	
6:00	
6:30	
7:00	
7:30	
8:00	
8:30	
9:00	
9:30	
10:00	
10:30	
11:00	
11:30	
P.M.	
12:00	
12:30	
1:00	
1:30	
2:00	
2:30	
3:00	
3:30	
4:00	
4:30	
5:00	
5:30	
6:00	
6:30	
7:00	
7:30	
8:00	
8:30	
9:00	
9:30	
10:00	
10:30	
11:00	

IDEAL DAILY SCHEDULE

Time	Activity (meal, exercise, or supplements)
A.M.	
5:30	
6:00	
6:30	
7:00	
7:30	
8:00	
8:30	
9:00	
9:30	
10:00	
10:30	
11:00	
11:30	
P.M.	
12:00	
12:30	
1:00	
1:30	
2:00	
2:30	
3:00	
3:30	
4:00	
4:30	
5:00	
5:30	
6:00	
6:30	
7:00	
7:30	
8:00	
8:30	
9:00	
9:30	
10:00	
10:30	
11:00	

APPENDIX

Notes regarding this gram counter:

1.   I have not included foods that I do not recommend you eat (such as pork, shellfish, bread, regular pasta, and so forth).

2. "Trace" means less than .5 or less than 2 percent of the RDA.

Grams of Everything counter

Food Name	Serving Size	Calories	Protein Grams	Carb Grams	Fats Grams	Fiber Grams
ACORN SQUASH						
(baked)	½ cup	60	1	15	trace	2.0
ALMONDS,						
sliced	1 cup	560	19	19	49	4.4
APPLE, raw	1 medium	80	0	15	trace	3.0
	1 large	125	0	31	1	5.0
APPLE JUICE						
(natural)	6 oz	76	0	19	0	0
APPLESAUCE						
(natural	½ cup	100	trace	22	0	na
APRICOTS, raw	3 medium	52	trace	12	trace	1.4
dried	2 oz	140	2	35	0	na
ARTICHOKE	1 medium	30	3	12	0	1.5
ARTICHOKE HEARTS						
frozen	3 oz	30	2	7	0	3.0
ASPARAGUS,						
fresh	4 spears	13	2	2	trace	.6
canned	½ cup	20	2	3	0	1.2
frozen	3.3 ounces	25	3	4	0	na
AVOCADO (Calif)	1 medium	306	4 or less	12	30	4.7
BANANA, raw	1 medium	100	1	27	1 or less	1.8
BARLEY, cooked	1 cup	193	4	44	1 or less	.4
BEANS, baked						
vegetarian	7 ¾ ounces	170	11	40	1	na
BEEF, bottom round	2.8 oz	175	25	0	8	0

Food Name	Serving Size	Calories	Protein Grams	Carb Grams	Fats Grams	Fiber Grams
BEEF, chuck blade	2.2 ounces	170	19	0	9	0
BEEF, ground (broiled)	3 ounces	230	21	0	16	0
BEEF, rib (roasted)	2.2 oz	150	17	0	9	0
BEEF, eye of round roasted)	2.6 oz	135	22	0	5	0
BEEF, sirloin steak broiled	2.5 oz	150	22	0	6	0
BEEF, canned corned	3 oz	185	22	0	10	0
BEEF, dried chipped	2.5 oz	145	24	0	4	0
BEETS, sliced						
cooked	1 cup	55	2	12	0	4
canned	½ cup	35	1	8	0	na
BLACKBERRIES	½ cup	37	less than 1	9	trace	3.3
BLUEBERRIES	½ cup	41	less than 1	10	trace	1.7
BLUEFISH (baked or broiled)	3 oz	140	21	0	4	0
BOK CHOY, cooked	1 cup	25	2	4	0	na
BOUILLON,						
Beef	1 cube	6	less than 1	1	less than 1	0
Chicken	1 cube	8	less than 1	1	less than 1	0
Onion	1 cube	8	less than 1	1	less than 1	0
BROCCOLI, fresh	1 cup	40	5	7	0	4.0
frozen	3.3 oz	30	3	5	0	3.0
BRUSSELS SPROUTS						
fresh	1 cup	55	7	10	1	7.0
frozen	3.3 oz	35	3	7	0	3.0
BULGAR WHEAT						
cooked	1 cup	152	6	34	trace	.6
BUTTER	1 tbsp	65	0	0	12	0
BUTTERMILK (1%)	1 cup	100	8	12	2	0
CABBAGE,						
raw	1 cup	16	1	4	trace	.8
cooked	1 cup	32	1	7	trace	1.0
Chinese, raw	1 cup	10	1	less than 2	trace	.8
CANTALOUPE	½	94	2	22	less than 1	2.1
CARROTS, raw	1	30	1	7	0	3.0
cooked	1 cup	50	1	11	0	5.0
frozen	3.3 oz	40	1	9	0	2.0
CASABA MELON	1 wedge	40	2	9	0	.8
CASHEWS	⅓ cup	260	8	14	21	2.5
CAULIFLOWER, raw	1 cup	25	3	5	trace	2.4
cooked	1 cup	30	3	5	trace	2.8
frozen	3.3 oz	25	2	5	0	2
CELERY	1 stalk	5	0	2	0	1
CHERRIES, fresh sour	1 cup	90	2	23	trace	.5
sweet	1 cup	104	2	26	less than 1	1.0
CHESTNUTS	⅓ cup	100	2	22	1	5.0
CHICKEN, dark meat	4 oz	232	31	0	11	0
CHICKEN, white meat	4 oz	196	35	0	5	0

Food Name	Serving Size	Calories	Protein Grams	Carb Grams	Fats Grams	Fiber Grams
CHICKEN, roasted with skin	4 oz	253	27	0	15	0
CHICK PEAS cooked	½ cup	110	6	17	0	3.0
canned	½ cup	77	4	12	1	3.2
CHILIES, green chopped	2 tbsp	7	0	1	less than 1	na
COD (broiled)	4 oz	109	23	0	1	0
CORN, fresh	1 cup	140	6	21	1	3
canned cream	½ cup	80	2	18	1	na
canned, kernel	½ cup	70	2	18	0	2
frozen	3.3 oz	80	3	20	1	2
COUSCOUS, cooked	½ cup	100	4	20	0	na
CRANBERRIES, raw	1 cup	100	2	26	trace	1.2
CRANBERRY JUICE, low-cal cocktail	6 oz	5	0	9	0	0
CUCUMBER, raw	1 cup	16	2	4	trace	1.0
CURRANTS	½ cup	200	2	53	0	2.0
DATES	1 cup	490	10	130	1	8.0
DUCK, roasted (skinless)	4 oz	228	27	0	13	0
EGG, whole	1 large	80	6	less than 1	5	0
white only	1	17	less than 4	trace	0	0
EGG SUBSTITUTE	¼ cup	60	6	3	3	0
EGGPLANT, boiled	1 cup	38	2	8	0	1
ENDIVE, raw	1 cup	10	less than 1	2	trace	.4
FLOUNDER, baked or broiled	3 oz	170	21	0	7	0
GARLIC	1 clove	4	0	1	0	.1
GRAPES	10	35	0	9	0	.4
GRAPEFRUIT	½	50	1	13	0	.3
GRAPEFRUIT JUICE unsweetened	8 oz	100	1	24	0	0
GREEN BEANS, cooked fresh	1 cup	30	2	7	0	2.2
frozen	3 oz	25	1	6	0	2
GREENS, beet	1 cup	25	2	5	0	na
GREENS, collard	1 cup	65	7	10	1	6.0
GREENS, dandelion	1 cup	35	2	7	1	na
GREENS, Mustard	1 cup	30	3	5	0	na
GREENS, turnip	1 cup	30	3	5	0	4.4
HALIBUT (baked) or broiled)	4 oz	159	30	0	3	0
HONEYDEW MELON	⅒	46	less than 1	8	trace	0
KALE fresh (boiled)	1 cup	45	2	7	1	1
KIDNEY BEANS, fresh, cooked	1 cup	220	na	40	1	10
canned	½ cup	90	7	20	less than 1	5.0
KUMQUAT	1 med	12	trace	3	0	.7
LAMB (lean), chop	1.7 oz	135	17	0	7	0
leg	2.6 oz	140	20	0	6	0

Food Name	Serving Size	Calories	Protein Grams	Carb Grams	Fats Grams	Fiber Grams
LEMON	1	20	1	6	0	0
LENTILS, cooked	1 cup	230	18	40	trace	.4
LETTUCE, Bibb	1 leaf	2	trace	trace	trace	.5
LETTUCE, Iceberg	½ head	35	less than 3	6	less than 1	2.7
LETTUCE, shredded	1 cup	10	less than 1	2	trace	.4
LIMA BEANS, cooked, dry	1 cup	260	12	49	1	7.2
frozen	3.3 oz	130	7	24	0	na
LIME	1	20	less than 1	7	1	.3
LOGANBERRIES	1 cup	90	1	22	1	4.3
MACKEREL (broiled)	3 oz	200	20	0	14	0
MANGO, fresh	1 cup	108	less than 1	28	trace	1.8
MILK, skim	1 cup	85	8	12	0	0
MUSHROOMS, fresh, sliced	1 cup	20	2	3	0	1.0
MUSTARD	1 Tbsp	10	1	1	1	0
NAVY BEANS, cooked	1 cup	220	24	41	1	6.9
NECTARINE	1	67	1	16	less than 1	2.2
OIL, olive	1 Tbsp	120	0	0	14	0
OIL, walnut	1 Tbsp	120	0	0	14	0
OKRA, fresh, cooked	10 pods	30	2	6	0	2.0
frozen	3.3 oz	30	2	7	0	na
OLIVES, green	4	20	0	trace	2	.4
OLIVES, ripe	4	20	0	trace	2	.4
ONION, white, chopped	1 cup	65	3	15	0	2.6
ONION, green, chopped	6	15	0	3	0	1.2
ORANGE	1	65	1	16	0	.6
ORANGE JUICE, fresh	6 oz	83	1	19	trace	.2
PAPAYA	1 cup	55	1	14	0	1.2
PARSLEY	1 tbsp.	2	trace	trace	trace	trace
PARSNIPS (boiled)	1 cup	100	2	23	1	4.2
PEACHES, fresh	1	39	less than 1	10	trace	1.4
dried	2 ounces	140	2	35	0	3.3
PEAR, fresh	1	100	1	25	trace	6
PEAS, fresh	1 cup	110	8	25	trace	6
canned (low sodium)	1/2 cup	50	4	11	0	3
frozen	3.3 oz	80	5	13	0	4
PEPPERS, red or green	1	20	less than 1	5	trace	1.2
PICKLE, bread & butter	1 oz	30	0	7	0	na
PICKLE, dill spears	1 oz	4	0	1	0	na
PICKLE, hamburger dill	1 oz	4	0	1	0	na
PIKE, Northern (broiled)	4 oz	128	28	0	1	0
PIMIENTO	1 oz	10	0	2	0	na
PINEAPPLE, fresh	1 cup	80	less than 1	22	less than 1	1.8
canned (unsweetened)	6 oz	100	0	25	0	na
PINTO BEANS	½ cup	117	7	22	trace	3.7
PLANTAIN	1	313	2	57	1	.9
PLUM, fresh	1	30	0	8	0	.4
POMPANO (broiled)	4 oz	239	26	0	14	0

Food Name	Serving Size	Calories	Protein Grams	Carb Grams	Fats Grams	Fiber Grams
POPCORN, plain	4 cups	140	3	17	7	3
PUMPKIN, cooked, mashed	½ cup	24	1	6	trace	4
PUMPKIN seeds	1 cup	90	0	22	0	na
QUAIL	1	125	24	0	4	0
RADISHES	10 med	10	0	2	trace	.2
RAISINS (natural)	3 oz	250	3	63	0	4
RASPBERRIES, black	1 cup	100	1	21	2	na
red	1 cup	70	1	17	less than 1	5.8
RED BEANS, canned	4 oz	112	5	18	2	5.5
RED SNAPPER (broiled)	4 oz	145	3	0	2	0
REFRIED BEANS, canned	4 oz	130	7	20	2	na
RICE, brown	½ cup	110	2	23	0	1.7
RICE, wild	1 cup	166	7	35	less than 1	2.4
ROCKFISH (broiled)	4 oz	140	27	0	2	0
RUTABAGA, fresh, cooked	1 cup	60	less than 2	14	trace	5.5
SALMON, broiled	4 oz	208	31	0	8	0
SALMON, canned pink	½ cup	160	20	0	7	0
SALMON, canned red	½ cup	180	21	0	9	na
SALMON, smoked	1 oz	50	5	0	3	0
SARDINES, canned						
in soy bean oil	1 can	380	19	na	34	0
SAUERKRAUT	1 oz	4	0	1	0	na
SCALLIONS	6	15	0	3	0	1.2
SOLE (baked or broiled)	4 oz	133	27	0	2	0
SPINACH, raw, chopped	1 cup	12	2	2	trace	1.4
fresh, cooked	1 cup	42	5	7	trace	4
canned, no salt	½ cup	25	2	4	0	na
frozen	3.3 oz	20	3	3	0	3
SQUASH, summer	1 cup	30	2	7	trace	2
Squash, winter	1 cup	130	3	32	1	6
STRAWBERRIES, fresh	1 cup	46	1	10	less than 1	3.8
SUNFLOWER seeds	1 oz	160	7	6	13	4.4
SWORDFISH, broiled	3 oz	140	24	0	6	0
TANGARINE	1	40	1	10	0	.3
TOFU (soybean cake)	4 oz	82	9	3	5	1.2
TOMATO, fresh	1	26	1	6	trace	1.6
canned, whole, no salt	4 oz	20	0	5	0	na
stewed, no salt	½ cup	35	2	8	0	na
TUNA, (albacore)						
canned in water	4 oz	144	32	0	1	0
TURKEY, light meat						
(skinless)	4 oz	200	37	0	4	0
TURKEY, dark meat	4 oz	233	35	0	9	0
TURNIP, cooked	1 cup	35	1	8	0	4.6
VEAL (broiled) lean cutlet	4 oz	250	31	0	12	0
loin chop	4 oz	235	39	0	8	0
VEGETABLES, mixed						
frozen	3.3 oz	100	2	11	5	2

Food Name	Serving Size	Calories	Protein Grams	Carb Grams	Fats Grams	Fiber Grams
VINEGAR	2 tbsp.	0	0	1	0	0
WALNUTS, chopped	½ cup	260	9	6	25	2.1
WATERCRESS	10 sprigs	3	less than 1	trace	trace	.6
WATERMELON	1 slice	150	3	35	2	1.9
WHITEFISH (smoked)	3 oz	175	24	0	1.05	0
YAM, cooked	½ cup	80	1	19	trace	na
ZUCCHINI, cooked	1 cup	22	2	5	0	1

BIBLIOGRAPHY

Hintermister, William. *How to Get Rid of Your Double Chin in Just Six Weeks.* 1982.

Sonberg, Lynn. *The Complete Nutrition Counter.* (New York: Berkley Books, 1993).

ABOUT THE AUTHOR

TED BROER is a university-trained biochemist, exercise physiologist, and licensed nutritionist. He holds a master's degree in business administration, and additional degrees in biology, chemistry and psychology. He has also completed extensive post-graduate work in the fields of nutrition and biochemistry. With more than a decade of clinical experience he has helped thousands lower their blood pressure, cholesterol, and body fat levels.

Broer has been featured on thousands of radio and television programs internationally and has spoken to approximately one million individuals at live seminars.

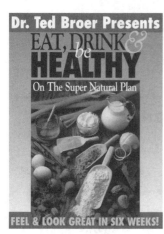

EAT, DRINK, AND BE HEALTHY TAPE PROGRAM
by Dr. Ted and Sharon Broer
Our six week program to optimal Health and Energy!

Tape 1: The Top Ten Foods Never to Eat

Tape 2: Forever Slim (Do's and Don'ts of Weight Loss)

Tape 3: Winning Choices for Your Health

Tape 4: Double Your Energy, Double Your Output

Tape 5: Simplifying the Supermarket Safari

Tape 6: Foods That Heal

Tape 7: Food Choices: Facts & Myths

Tape 8: Answers to Our Most Frequently Asked Questions.

Plus reports on: ADD, Hypertension, Cancer, Diabetes, Depression, and Prostate Problems.

FOREVER FIT: AT 20, 30, 40, AND BEYOND TAPE SERIES
by Dr. Ted Broer
Lose Weight* Feel Great* Fitness/Health Series
Our latest, up-to-date series on Health, Nutrition, Sports Medicine, and exercise!

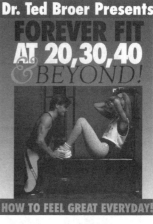

Tape 1: Fat Loss, Not Weight Loss—The Key to Looking Great! Hormones and How They Control the Body.

Tape 2: Exercise—Its Role in Burning Fat/Lean Muscle Mass—What Types & How much

Tape 3: Trace Minerals, Vitamin Supplements, Fatty Acids/Join Repair and Arthritis

Tape 4: Artificial Sweeteners/Chemicals and Foods in Our Environment to Avoid

Tape 5: Chronic Fatigue Syndrome, Yeast Infection, Hypoglycemia, and Your Immune System

Tape 6: Constipation, the Colon, and Your Health

Tape 7: Fasting: The Physical & Spiritual Benefits

Tape 8: Water: Use a Filter or Be a Filter/Why You Absorb As Many Toxins in One Hot Shower as If You Had Drunk 8 Glasses of Contaminated Water.

Plus reports on: Nutrasweet, Constipation, Eating for body fat loss, Yeast infections, Epstein-Barr, and Chronic Fatigue Syndrome

TO ORDER CALL 1-800-726-1834

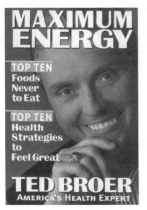

MAXIMUM ENERGY BOOK
by Dr. Ted Broer

- The Top Ten Foods Never to Eat!
- The Top Ten Health Strategies for Maximum Energy!
- Double your energy in 30 days with the right choices in this insightful book!

MAXIMUM ENERGY COOKBOOK
by Sharon Broer

A Health Guide to Survive! This book is an ideal gift for loved ones.

It includes:

- Back to basics recipes
- Infant, toddler, & children's diet
- Holiday Recipes
- Drinks, shakes, and coolers
- Fruit, vegetables, grains, and meat recipes
- Stress avoidance, exercise, water, goat's milk, and more . . .

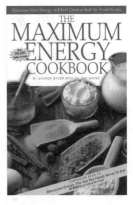

TRAIN UP YOUR CHILDREN IN THE WAY THEY SHOULD EAT
The Ultimate childrens program
A must for every concerned parent
by Sharon Broer

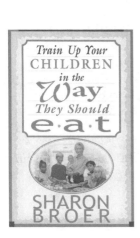

- Ensure the good health of your unborn baby.
- Nourish the infant and toddler so they can thrive.
- Protect and enhance the all-important immune systems of your children.
- Fuel active minds and bodies for complete physical and mental growth.
- Learn what your pediatrician won't tell you about nutrition and your child's health
- Stop serving the beverage that's more toxic than lead!
- No Ritalin
- No Ear infection
- No Allergies

EAT, DRINK AND BE HEALTHY EXERCISE VIDEOS

by Dr. Broer
A scientific Approach to Athletic Conditioning and Proper Nutrition.
It Includes:
- Non Impact Training
- Lean Muscle Growth & Fat Loss in 6 Weeks
- For Men and Women of all ages
- Three tape series for Men or Women - 6 total tapes
- Lifetime warranty on videos

UNDERSTANDING GOD'S DIETARY PRINCIPLES TAPE SERIES

This one answers all the Biblical Nutrition Questions
by Dr. Broer
Tape 1: How God's Dietary Principles Relate to Us
Tape 2: In Depth Scriptural Overview
Tape 3: How to Break the Dietary Curses of Degenerative Disease

HYPOGLYCEMIA: A SENSIBLE APPROACH TAPE SERIES

by Dr. Broer
Tape 1: Sugar & Controlling Hypoglycemia
Tape 2: Sugar and the American Sweet Tooth
Tape 3: What has Happened to Our Health?
If you have it, you need this series.

NUTRITION AND YOUR HEALTHY HEART TAPE SERIES

by Dr. Broer
Tape 1: Preventing Heart Disease
Tape 2: Exercising the Smart Way
Tape 3: Stress and Your Health
Learn how to keep this critical organ in top shape.

NATURAL COOKING FOR THE HOLIDAYS TAPE SERIES

by Sharon Broer
Tape 1: Using Meat Replacements and Grains
Tape 2: Holiday Meal Planning
Tape 3: Sugar Replacements and Holiday Desserts
For those who ask: "Where do I start?"

BREAKING THE DIETARY CURSES OF CANCER TAPE SERIES

by Dr. Broer
Tape 1: Cancer Prevention
Tape 2: The Benefits of Fasting
Tape 3: Fiber and a Healthy Colon
Tape 4: God's Dietary Principles
Tape 5: Clean & Unclean Foods
The nation's 2nd largest killer can be prevented.

HELPING YOUR FAMILY MAKE DIETARY CHANGES TAPE SERIES

by Dr. Ted and Sharon Broer
Tape 1: Fiber & Food Preparation
Tape 2: Healthy Food Substitutes
Tape 3: Attitudes on Nutrition
This one makes it easy!

PREVENTING ARTHRITIS AND OSTEOPOROSIS TAPE SERIES

by Dr. Broer
Tape 1: Arthritis and Osteoporosis
Tape 2: The Importance of Calcium
Tape 3: Is Supplementation Necessary?
It's easier to prevent!

TRAIN UP A CHILD IN THE WAY HE SHOULD EAT TAPE SERIES

by Sharon Broer
Tape 1: Prenatal Nutrition
Tape 2: Infant & Toddler Nutrition
Tape 3: A Child's Diet
A must for those with children.

PLEASE CALL 1-800-726-1834 FOR CURRENT PRICES AND SPECIALS